WITH TWO SOULS

For our families; those we were lucky enough to be given, and those we were lucky enough to choose. Especially our parents, Amanda and Chris, and Askalech and Kidane, and our children, Mesmora, Natnael, Raphael and Ivy.

WITH TWO SOULS

Two midwives' recollections of love, life, birth,
and death in rural Ethiopia

Indie McDowell & Atsede Kidane

With Two Souls: Two midwives' recollections of love, life, birth, and death in rural Ethiopia

First published by Pinter & Martin 2022

ISBN 978-1-78066-770-6
Also available as ebook

British Library Cataloguing-in-Publication Data
A catalogue record for this book is available from the British Library.

Set in Dante

Printed and bound in the UK by Severn

Pinter & Martin Ltd
6 Effra Parade
London SW2 1PS

pinterandmartin.com

Contents

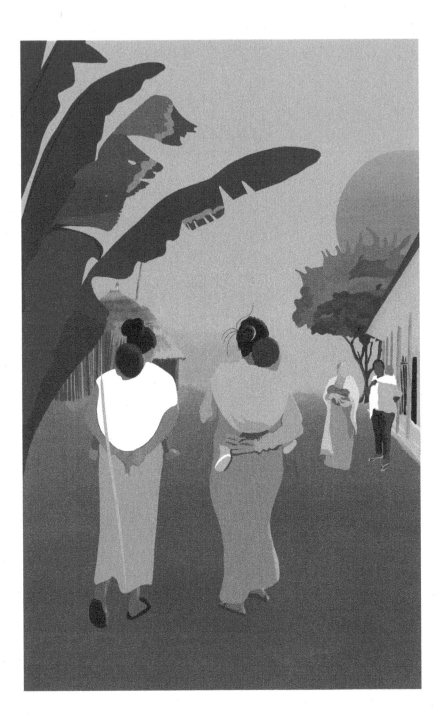

Preface

The moments and memories recounted here are from the years Atsede and Indie have spent working together in the highlands of Gurage Zone, Ethiopia, in a small market town called Gubrye. The town itself has existed for only a handful of years longer than their Clinic, but the villages that surround it are ancient and have been lived in for generations, with many ways of life the same now as they were then. Atsede was born in one such village, Cesar Soast, and spent much of her childhood living with her eldest sister in another, Buchachj.

Atsede and Indie first met in the summer of 2016, when Indie joined the staff at Attat Hospital, run by the Medical Missionary Sisters, just a stone's throw from Cesar Soast, where Atsede led the midwifery services. For the next couple of years they were rarely apart, working together through thousands of hours and thousands of births. On Valentine's Day in 2018, Atsede's eldest son, Mesmora, was born in the same operating theatre where she had spent so much time as a midwife assisting the surgeons with caesareans. On that same day, Indie completed her final shift as a midwife at the hospital. As well as motherhood for Atsede, together she and Indie had another new adventure to embark on…

In the summer of 2018, after months of planning, fundraising, and building, and following the end of Atsede's *chyne* (postnatal period), the doors to their own Clinic were, at last, thrown open. Atsede and Indie began welcoming women into the Maternal and Child Health Outpatients Rooms, assisting with births in the Birth

Room, and treating patients in the Emergency Room.

A handful of months later, in spring 2019, Indie's son Raphael was born, with Atsede as her midwife. In spring 2021, Atsede's second son, Natnael, was born, with Indie as her midwife. The three boys have grown up together, as much like brothers as any related by blood. In the weeks and months before and between these births, Atsede and Indie have continued to work side-by-side at the Clinic, every day and night of the week except Sunday, in theory. In practice, though, they often work on Sunday too, simply dressed in their white church dresses, their *tibab*, instead of their white midwifery gowns.

Indie returns to England twice a year, in the summer and in the winter, to see her family there and to fundraise for the Clinic. Atsede has also spent the summer of the last five years attending university to gain her Bachelor's degree. She graduated in the summer of 2021 with a First, a remarkable achievement for a girl who learnt to write with sticks in the mud and read with the old medication packages her father brought home from the hospital.

This book is a tribute to the births, deaths, loves, losses, friendships, and fortitude shared by all of those who have walked into the lives of Atsede and Indie over the last six years, and has been written to capture the triumphs and tragedies of the extraordinary profession that is midwifery.

Introduction

Indie

The disjointed colours and sounds, the vague awareness that I was in a surgical operating theatre without being entirely sure as to why, but most of all the deep regret that I would die here, in Africa, and my family wouldn't know. There was a shocking finality to believing that death was approaching. I wasn't ready, I didn't want to die, I wanted to get up, get out, as far and as fast as I could. Instead, the blackness at the edge of my vision grew, and I was slowly sinking into it. Unable to understand any more, I let go, and disappeared, dissolving into a hundred thousand pieces.

Then, blinking, everything blurry, and seeing an IV stand, trying to comprehend that it led to my hand, slowly putting together the puzzle pieces. I was alive, of that much I was sure, but little else made sense. Voices talking next to me, voices I knew but couldn't place, and yet, somehow, just hearing them I was reassured. A hand, subconsciously and tenderly smoothing out a minute wrinkle in the surgical gown thrown across me, then resting gently against my own, a familiar, comfortable weight. But it was all too confusing, so back to sleep.

Time passes, but minutes or hours, I don't know. Again, seeing the IV. If I concentrate just on that, I feel calmer. Why would I feel calmer? Why do I know what an IV is? Why am I watching it and calculating the drop rate? Oh, I'm a midwife. I think about that for a while, turning it over in my mind. I know about IVs because I'm a midwife. I've sited a thousand, then started a bag of oxytocin infusion just like this. For women having babies. Babies. My baby!

Suddenly, in an instant, the mist lifts and I remember everything. The long labour, the bumpy *bajaj* ride to the hospital when I hadn't progressed in hours, the birth of my tiny son, and then the bleeding which wouldn't stop. With the return of reality, I turned to the voices, smiling, relieved, knowing now exactly who they were. I tried to focus on Selam and Atsede, keeping vigil, before my eyelids became too heavy, and once more, the oblivion of unconsciousness beckoned.

Nestled into the crook of Selam's arms, his big eyes taking it all in, a tiny fist in his mouth, was my son. Next to them, on the slightly broken chair that left its occupant slanted at an angle, was Atsede. It was her hand that came to my chest to check I wasn't cold, and to my wrist to check my pulse. Satisfied that, at last, all was well, Atsede settled back, propping her feet up on the bars of the theatre trolley on which I was lying and, turning to Selam, continued their conversation about the goats and the gardens. My eyes closed, and drifting in and out of awareness, I let their words wash over me, the mundanity of the topics and their casual tone answering the question I want to ask but can't construct the words for: 'Is my baby okay?'

Five years ago, when I first stepped off the plane onto the tarmac at Bole Airport, Addis Ababa, I never imagined my life would go this way. It was a very Ethiopian dawn, still chilled from the night-time mountain air, with taxi drivers gathered together stamping their feet and blowing on cold hands, waiting for passengers like me to collect their bags and head out into the city, where the fruit vendors already lined the roads with colourful baskets of mangoes, bananas, oranges, and papaya arranged on the pavement in front of them, and long, purple sugar canes stacked up beside them. Even at this time, the infamous Addis traffic was starting, with the ubiquitous blue Lada taxis nosing their way through impossible spaces between worn, old, white minibuses blaring loud music and big, black 4x4s. Weaving alongside, the motorbikes and pedestrians: students, with their uniforms and books and lunch tins, laughing and calling to friends emerging from alleyways on their way to school, office workers wearing suits and trainers, worshippers from the churches scattered across the city, white, woven *netela* scarves with brightly coloured borders tucked over their heads and thrown over one shoulder.

It is a city where chaos reigns, a city of contradictions. On the one hand, explosive growth and development, 'the hub of Africa', home to the headquarters of many of global multinationals. On the other, the beggars dressed in rags, desperately trying to survive on what little they can scrape together, sleeping rough with nothing between them and the pollution, the fumes, the weather. I would quickly come to understand that while being poor is hard anywhere, the character of poverty in the cities is very different from that in the countryside. Far more difficult, more lonely, more dangerous.

Thankfully, I was heading away from the madness, and as I made my way down the Arrivals ramp, I sought out Deriba, the driver from the hospital that would be my home for the next year. I found him, or rather he found me, and chatting amiably about nothing and everything we slowly wound our way through the city and out into the countryside, stopping only to pick up glistening watermelons from a wooden cart balanced against its donkey.

Lulled by the road, tarmac now, though only recently, and the vista of swaying *tef* crop and blue-hued mountains, I rested my head back against the seat and mused on what was to come. I knew the hospital, having spent several months working there the previous year, and I was looking forward to getting back to it. But I was nervous too, knowing the challenges that were coming.

What I didn't know then was how fundamentally it would change me, bearing witness to life and death every day. I didn't know that my understanding of what matters would shift, that I would learn not only how to save someone, but also how not to. I didn't know that Atsede, with her gentle, self-deprecating humour and quiet acceptance of both the challenges and triumphs of life, so typical of the Gurage women, would irrevocably change the course of my life, and that her lessons of love and laughter and friendship, of impossible choices and unwavering faith, would be taught not only in the busy wards of the hospital, but also in the cool, peaceful rooms of our own medical clinic and birth centre.

I'm delighted to say that the story didn't end with the birth of my son, and the ketamine that had induced my certainty of impending death soon wore off. Though woozy and aching, and feeling the effects of a significant blood loss, when the warm little bundle was placed in my arms, and nuzzling for a feed, I could hardly believe that such an amazing baby could be mine. Three years later, the feeling hasn't faded.

Practising as a midwife in rural Ethiopia has been quite the experience. Raising a baby in rural Ethiopia has been quite the experience. The last five years have been quite the experience. While I've missed my family, and at times yearned for them to see my son as he grows, this is a part of the world where the village that it takes to raise a child is very present. To be part of it has been such a privilege, and Raphael can be as proud of his belonging here as of his English, and Colombian, heritage.

Atsede

The pale wood of the heavy door to the theatre swung towards me, suddenly separating me from her. For the first time in my decade as a midwife I couldn't face going into an operation with a woman in my care. Because this wasn't just a woman, this was Indie. Indie, the first one to hold my son. Indie, who washed my birthing clothes by hand, as I would soon be washing hers, who tried to braid my hair as I recovered from my caesarean a year ago. The braids fell out the first time she tried, much to everyone's amusement, but by the fourth attempt they lasted three weeks. She was my closest friend, related by love if not by blood. We lived together, opened the clinic and birth centre together, laughed together, saved lives and lost lives. And now I stood, on the wrong side of the door, anxious and upset, second guessing and questioning every decision I had made over the last 11 hours. Should I have brought her to the hospital sooner? Should I have insisted she went back to England for her birth?

A quiet, sighing cry caught my attention, and I looked over to Selam. Her head was bent over the warm bundle stirring in her arms, a brown finger caressing a white cheek with love and gentle reassurance. Indie's son was beautiful, with big, almond-shaped eyes, navy for now but which would soon lighten to match exactly the blue of the endless *berga* – summer – skies. Settling under Selam's touch and murmurings, his eyes blinked, slowly, heavily, and, yawning, he gave in to sleep again. My heart skipped, loving him almost as much as I loved my own son, Mesmora. Then muffled voices from behind the door, and a wave of fear passed over me once more.

An hour later though, those feelings had dissipated completely. While Indie's birth story was different than she'd imagined, than we'd both imagined, this moment remained the same. A breathtaking, life-affirming instant in time when the world stood still. As I stood with my arm at her waist, and Selam placed Raphael in her arms, there were tears in all of our eyes. They had soon turned to laughter, though, as Selam and I watched Indie try not to show her discomfort as the older women among the staff came to see the new baby, making a *pthew-pthew* sound, almost, but not quite, spitting over his head, accompanied by heartfelt *'yitenwe'*, a combination of moves intended to protect against evil and attract blessing. It was a tradition I knew she didn't understand; even with Mesmora in her arms she had had to stop herself from flinching every time it happened. To her credit, though, and pointedly not acknowledging the smirking faces of Selam and I, she looked each woman in the eye and thanked them, the gratitude in her voice for their gesture genuine.

This story, our story, has a definite place where it all started for Indie. The day she stepped off the plane, and drove all those hours to the hospital. For me though, I can't decide. Did it start during those months I stayed with the Medical Missionary Sisters in their convent attached to the hospital, wondering whether I would lead the life of a novitiate and then nurse-nun? Or perhaps when I signed the agreement that would see me train as a midwife? Or, maybe, it was far earlier in my life, watching my father dress carefully every morning before walking several kilometres through airy eucalyptus forests to his position as a nurse's aide. In any case, I'm sure it was all of those moments, and many more, that combined to bring me to where I am today, sitting in the white-tiled rooms of Atsede Clinic, named for me but as much Indie's as mine, looking out of the window at the bright red flowers of the bottle-brush trees, listening to the sounds of my sons, and Indie's, giggling together as they plot to throw handfuls of water over the nurses, while in the room with me is a young woman, abdomen swollen with her baby, groaning through the contractions that will soon see her newborn daughter delivered into my hands.

It was something I could never have imagined, my own clinic. But then again, so much of midwifery has been unimaginable until it happens. So much of life. Three years we've been open now, treating thousands of patients and guiding women through hundreds of births. The stories we've written about here, those ending in both triumph and tragedy, represent only a handful of those I've been a part of, and I could fill shelves with the moments I've seen. I didn't believe Indie when she first told me we would write a book. I couldn't understand who would want to read it. But then Indie explained that these stories deserve to be told, even if they are only read by one person. Because just one person can make a difference. In the same way that that one midwife, caring for that one woman, does in that one moment in time. *Tibetib*, drop by drop, so that saying goes. The impact of just one seemingly insignificant instant is unknown, with ripples out far beyond where we can see.

Nowhere are women laid bare like in the birthing room. It is, at the same time, the most ordinary and extraordinary experience. And it links every human who is, or who has ever been, or will ever be, alive. There is terrible fighting in my country at the moment, bringing so much sadness and so much heartache. But the differences people think exist between us fade away in the birth room. No matter the colour of your skin, the faith in your heart, the thoughts in your mind, there is this one thread of experience that links us all.

And it is the midwives who stand there through it. That's the other reason Indie gave for why we should do this. For midwives. Indie could come to Ethiopia, with languages she didn't speak, and cultures she didn't understand, and find it her home, because there is a connection that exists between midwives. As with all professions, there are those who are lost, but no midwife starts their training without a desire to hold the hand of a woman through her pregnancy and birth. For centuries, midwives were cast not as the protagonists in guarding birth, but as the villains. I've long wondered about this, about why people were so afraid of us. All I can think is that it must be to do with fear. Of the power we hold in our hands and our hearts. You can't be a midwife without a fortitude that would put any tree withstanding the storms to shame, or a determination that could rival a river wanting to reach the ocean, or the resilience of the yellow *meskel* flower that blooms again and again, in times of deluge and times of drought.

We understand the secrets of women, the strength of their bodies and of their minds. We see things that no one else will ever be privileged enough to see, the first look between a mother and her baby, the gentle hand of a sister on the arm of a labouring woman, giving courage with just a touch. We make decisions that no one should ever have to make, whether to save a life or whether not to. So perhaps Indie was right: these stories deserve to be told. I hope you take something from reading them.

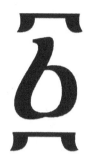

1

Melele

Indie

'Wait', I held out a gloved hand, the blue latex glowing luminescent in the soft, flickering candlelight, 'are you sure that's necessary?' I had seen Atsede reaching for the aluminium tin containing, among other instruments, the episiotomy scissors. It was cold and dark, the electricity having gone sometime in the early hours, and we were on night duty. It had been a full, satisfying shift so far, with several new babies adding their lusty voices to the world, and just as many happy, exhausted mothers snuggling newborns close and guiding little mouths to their breasts to suckle. We'd taken it in turns to help with the births, at least until I was called away for a caesarean in my role as neonatal lead, and had to leave the ward in Atsede's very capable hands. In the end, I wasn't really needed in theatre: the baby whose slowing growth and weight had worried the surgeons came out crying with all his might. I stayed long enough to help with the paperwork, and then, with the sweet, solemn-eyed baby tucked up with his mother, I took off my colourful theatre cap and mask, slipped them into my scrub pocket, and wandered back along the walkway to the delivery room.

Hours earlier, it had been the beating heart of the hospital, a semi-covered corridor stretching from the isolation rooms at one end up to the outpatients department at the other. Women in colourful dresses with gaudy scarves bound around their hair sat along the benches, bouncing young children with bandaged hands or feet or heads, or talking to relatives and friends holding on to makeshift drip stands. The nurses flittered around them, the pockets of their white gowns full with gauze and stethoscopes and packets of medication, occasionally shouting after the monkeys that swung over the rooftops and through the trees, trying to steal bits of fruit and bread from the visitors. Not so at this time of night, when instead of the noise and movement of life, still darkness cloaked everything, with just the glow of the gas-fed hurricane lanterns placed by the guards at the doorways so that the night staff could see where they were going.

Shivering into the air, and nodding to the new, and soon to be new, fathers sitting and dozing on the benches, I headed back inside, pausing to change shoes, take a sip of sweet, spiced tea, and wipe the woman's name off the high-risk list. Standing surveying the labour ward boards, and making sure I had a good idea of what was going on with medicines, blood pressure checks, and a thousand other things that were part of ensuring the women and their babies remained safe, I heard Atsede talking in soft, encouraging tones behind the curtains pulled around the furthest of the four beds. A glance at the stacks of notes on the desk told me what was going on. It was the beautiful, elegant young woman with dark, shimmering skin the colour of mahogany who came from the south. With her facial tattoos, unusual hairstyle and decorative beads, Melele was an exotic and mesmerising figure, keeping her graceful walk with her head held high even through her strong contractions. She had progressed well, and the sweat beading lightly on her hairline suggested it might almost be time.

This was her first pregnancy, and everything was going as expected through her labour, with the baby moving down well, and Melele staying calm and collected. I couldn't shake the feeling that Atsede's decision to perform an episiotomy would only disrupt the delicate balance that had settled around Melele, and disturb her focus, interrupting the concentration that had moved her baby so effectively this far. I didn't understand why it was needed either; I couldn't see the indication. Talking quietly and carefully so as not to disturb Melele, I challenged Atsede's judgement, calling on my training in the UK and the papers I'd read considering routine episiotomy in primiparous (first time) women, and pointing out how it was now considered an unnecessary intervention, often doing more harm than good. Atsede calmly surveyed me, but there was a steely edge to her look. I knew her well enough to understand that she didn't like that I had questioned her decision.

'But', she asked, just as quietly and carefully, 'How much of your research was done on women like us? In places like this? Under circumstances like ours?' Atsede's eyes flicked to mine, but her concentration remained on Melele, one hand resting gently on the swell of her stomach, assessing the contractions almost without thinking about it, the other with a pen poised to record her findings on the partograph, the chart tracking a labour and delivery, with warning lines indicating if things were taking too long, open on the stainless steel, wheeled table.

Frowning to myself, caught unaware, I thought about Atsede's questions as I absentmindedly twisted the head of my stethoscope backwards and forwards, waiting until the wave of contraction that had just come over Melele subsided before checking her blood pressure. It was true. All the studies and evidence and best practice recommendations I knew about and talked of so surely came from far away, from white-tiled birth centres with trolleys always well stocked with towels and sheets, or from brightly lit delivery wards with vases of flowers sitting on desktops next to thank you cards and charity collection pots. They didn't come from here, where women sleep with their newborns on cardboard on the floor because all the beds are taken, and where buckets are placed strategically to catch the rain that oftentimes drips through the corrugated iron roof. Conceding the truth of her questions, in that moment I realised that as much as she had taught me already, Atsede still had many lessons left.

'Will you tell me about it?' It was some time later, after Melele was settled into a corner of the postnatal room, her new daughter sleeping peacefully beside her. This was my acknowledgement to Atsede that I, like midwives everywhere, wanted to know about anything that can help women in my care. She knew me well enough to understand that it also served as an apology for doubting her. Her face softened as she turned to me, smiling with understanding as her treacle-coloured eyes met mine. And just like that, the space between us that had been there while we finished caring for Melele closed, and we were once again facing the night together rather than at odds.

Atsede spoke at length afterwards, as we continued to wash the birth kits we had used that night. In a place where medical equipment was hard to come by, nothing was single use. The autoclave standing on a low table in the corner next to the nurses' desk provided a near-constant background hum as it heated the metal instruments to a temperature bacteria couldn't survive. Next to it sat the camping stove, with a metal tray full of water boiling the rubber components that couldn't survive it either, but still needed sterilising. While passing the clamps and scissors between buckets of bleach, water and soap, the first stage of their cleaning, I heard of the complicated lacerations that Atsede had seen and repaired, of the women with third- and fourth-degree tears that had broken down and had to be debrided, with necrotic tissue cut away before being sutured again, of the few women over the last several years who had died from sepsis or septicaemia. The tearing of the soft tissues of the birth canal isn't unique to women here, with almost 80% of women having their first babies expected to experience something of this.

That said, there are differences between the women here and the women elsewhere, not just in the standards of healthcare available, but also as a result of one particular practice: female circumcision. While reports claim that the practice is coming to an end, and that does seem to be the case in the urban areas, out here over 95% of women of childbearing age have had some form of modification. It is the same in the further reaches of the country, stretching across the borders into Somalia in the east, Djibouti and Sudan in the north and west, and Kenya to the south. Among some ethnic groups, the Afar and the Harari, this is the most extreme form of circumcision, known in places as *sunna,* pharaonic, or more formally within WHO documents, Type III. In essence, this is the removal of all labial tissue to leave just a small, penny-sized opening to allow urination and menstruation and, later, intercourse. The physical effects of such a circumcision are potentially life-threatening, from complicated infections to terrible pain. In a sense, the women of Gurage Zone are luckier. Type III circumcision has never been practised, and was even, until recently, largely unheard of. At the hospital, it was only seen when women visiting from the practising communities were caught unawares by pregnancies progressing to birth earlier than expected.

Where women have undergone circumcision, elsewhere known

as cutting, the musculature and skin of the perineum just doesn't behave as it would have normally. Although Type II circumcision doesn't directly affect the perineum, the area where episiotomies are performed, a consideration of the anatomy can shed some light. The muscles of the perineal body aren't simply linear, stretching from left to right. Instead, there is a complex interplay between the perineal muscles. Together, they form a delicate, interconnected, neurovascular web that facilitates the final moments of birth. Disrupt any one part of that, and it will unbalance the whole, which is exactly what is happening with a woman who has undergone circumcision. The removal of the labia minora and the clitoris irreversibly changes the anatomy forever. After all, interfering with natural physiology is bound to leave its mark. Without the stretch and the give, but instead with tight and unforgiving scar tissue, tears are unpredictable, splintering and fracturing along invisible fault lines. These may be because of the remnants of incomplete removal of the labia, the dissection away of too much tissue, or the formation of tough, white scars with little flexibility, all of which can be responsible for redistributing the force of the head moving through in ways that wouldn't happen with uncircumcised women.

'It's not just the tearing that is cause for concern', Atsede was saying, keen for me to understand, 'But the days and weeks afterwards'. It was true: in rural Ethiopia, women often go home to rooms and mattresses not clean enough to keep infection at bay. The water supplies are unreliable, compounding the problems. Far from health facilities, and without any postnatal visits to ensure the wound is healing, women go on to experience great pain and terrible infections.

'What I have seen making this better,' Atsede explained, 'is an episiotomy. That way, I know how and where the laceration is, and I know I can repair it well'. The last words of her statement I would certainly not refute. A right medio-lateral episiotomy (the customary approach in Ethiopia) will always be performed the same way, at the same angle, to the same depth. It is an intervention the midwives are taught in detail, witness throughout their training, and have performed countless times. It is quick and efficient and, despite the lack of pain relief, from experience I would argue largely unnoticed with the timing matching a peak of a contraction and the concentrated effort on pushing. The baby is born, and the subsequent repair can be carried out. Again, given there is often no pain relief available, with what little lidocaine there is saved for the emergency rooms and operating theatres, having a midwife trying to find the missing edges of torn tissues to align is less than desirable. On the other hand, the practised ease and artistry of watching the midwives bring together an episiotomy, with nothing more than the faintest hairline scar indicating there was ever a gaping assault on the delicate tissues in the first place, leaves no doubt as to the expertise of their repairs. Instead of trying to handle a configuration of torn tissues that they may not have seen before, the midwife can quickly, effectively, and almost with thinking, suture an episiotomy before the women have too much time to process the sharp sting of a needle. How many times had I seen Atsede do just this?

Like so many other moments during my hours attending birthing women, I wondered how to decide what was best. If performing an episiotomy on 10 women prevents one woman from a difficult tear and all the complications that might come with it, does that mean it's worth it? And moreover, who has the power and heavy responsibility to make such a call? I mulled over these questions as I washed down the bed Melele had used, with Atsede watching me half-amused, half-exasperated that I still couldn't quite come to terms with the need for such a painful, invasive procedure.

It wasn't that I'd found an answer when my introspective theorising on the natures of medical choices quickly ceased, but instead that the calm of the dawn hours was interrupted by a trolley being wheeled, with haste, into the delivery room. Recumbent on it was a young girl, hardly old enough to be away from home, let alone wed and pregnant, with a distended belly and deep, dark shadows under exhausted eyes. Pushing the trolley was one of the nurses from the Emergency Room, his forehead creased with worry, his hands nervously groping for a hastily written referral. His relief at seeing Atsede and I ready to take over was palpable. The scrap of paper that served as her medical, surgical, and obstetric history was folded tight in the fist of a slightly older girl whose resemblance to the almost unconscious patient left little doubt that she was her sister.

'Okay, bring her here. What is it? What's going on?' Atsede's sure, confident demeanour had a settling effect on the room. Along with Kidist, the sister keeping vigil, I felt myself breathe a little easier. Atsede was the best midwife in this part of the country to handle emergencies. I'd worked alongside her often enough to know.

The sad tale came out, interrupted occasionally by Atsede and myself pressing for details. It was a story we'd unfortunately heard before, albeit with slight differences here and there. We were right in our suspicions though. Tsigey, the patient, was really too young to be here. Her sister couldn't give a specific age – women rarely can – but believed Tsigey was somewhere between 12 and 14. At this I started to open my mouth to comment, but was hushed by a slight shake of the head by Atsede. Now was not the time. Later I was to learn that among the Kembatta, as well as other of the many ethnic groups that make up Ethiopia, such young brides were not uncommon.

Tsigey had gone into labour three days ago. At this Atsede and I both stopped Kidist for clarification. Three days? Was she sure it was that long? Kidist nodded, unaware of our realisation at that point that we knew how this would end. For three endless days and wearying nights, Tsigey had walked and squatted and cried, willing and praying for her baby to be delivered. As the hours passed, she, and her sisters and mother slowly realised that all was not well, and Tsigey wasn't experiencing birth the way others in the village had.

Finally, near collapse as the sun set on yet another day, Kidist managed to convince Tsigey and her husband that they had to get to the hospital. Tracking down several young men who could trade off carrying Tsigey on a litter took a while, but eventually enough turned up. The villages lie in the foothills of the Rift Valley mountains, with deep furrows gouged out of well-trodden tracks, a result of the two months of torrential *keremt* rains that bring life-giving water to the otherwise dry grounds. The rugged terrain makes many villages inaccessible to all but the toughest of vehicles, which are few and far between in any case. Moving around is done on foot, by donkey-cart, or, occasionally, by motorbike. For those too unwell to make a journey themselves, boughs of eucalyptus bound with vines, strips of old cloth, bits of old rubber tyres, almost anything that can be knotted and tied, are used as a litter, resting on the shoulders of men who carry their charge, often covered in thick blankets, to the nearest health facility.

This had been the case for Tsigey. By the time her litter-bearers reached us, there was nothing we could do for the baby, who had likely succumbed some hours before. Instead, it was Tsigey whose life we feared for. Having heard enough, Atsede took over. We transferred a now unconscious Tsigey to one of the delivery beds, pulled the curtains closed, and asked Kidist to give us a few moments. It's difficult to see someone you love on the receiving end of the management of an obstetric emergency. I went through the initial steps, making sure Tsigey was breathing, moving the oxygen concentrator from the obstetric operating theatre to the bedside just in case, starting IVs in both her hands with bags of fluid hung up high to help flush the big dose of prophylactic antibiotics through her veins and around her body, and placing a catheter into her bladder to help relieve the pressure of urine that couldn't be naturally passed given the position of the baby's head.

While Kidist was talking us through her sister's devastating few days, Atsede had been using her battered but trusted pinard to try and find a heartbeat. I'd been watching every now and again, with sad dismay but without surprise, as Atsede's hands glided over Tsigey's stomach, finding the landmarks of her baby's head, bottom, and back, and moving the pinard from one place to another, trying to hear the whooshing thud of a heartbeat. As we had expected, there wasn't one, but even knowing that was likely to be the case didn't assuage the moment of sorrow we couldn't help but feel. It had just been too many hours, too many days. A baby can't survive the pressure of contractions for that long; it's too hard on their tiny body, with the precious oxygen needed to survive temporarily reduced with each one. Usually, there is rest enough for the levels in the baby's blood to recover, and for the build-up of carbon dioxide to be filtered out by the miraculous placenta. Over time, though, the ability of the baby to compensate, and therefore live, faces just one too many assaults, getting less and less effective with each challenge until, finally, it isn't enough. As a midwife in the UK, it's possible to watch this decline in the biophysical numbers, with foetal scalp sampling allowing a tiny amount of the baby's blood to be taken from the top of their head and run through an analysing machine. The results show the coping mechanisms in action: the acidity of the blood and the attempt by the body to resolve this by flooding the cells with hydrogen ions to neutralise. Interventions are swift, with a theatre team ready for an emergency 'Cat 1' caesarean section, and a baby delivered into the waiting hands of a neonatal crash team. For Tsigey, this is impossible even to imagine. Her baby would have produced more and more hydrogen as the acid-base balance became more and more deranged until finally, there was nothing more to do.

With this knowledge, and a muffled silence through the pinard, while I was getting Tsigey stabilised Atsede had gone to wake Dr Rita, the obstetrician/gynaecologist and Catholic missionary nun who single-handedly keeps the hospital running with an inimitable energy and indomitable will. With a little over twenty years of experience working here in Ethiopia, and despite her unassuming ways, my faith in Dr Rita's ability to handle almost any critical situation is absolute. Indeed, I have Dr Rita to thank not only for teaching me so many essential lessons in midwifery, and in life, but for the safe arrival of my own son into the world, and for seeing me through the subsequent bleeding.

Minutes later, Dr Rita followed Atsede through the sluice room doors, pulling on a white coat and listening intently as she did so. Despite just having been woken, she was very much in control, and focused on saving the life of a birthing woman in crisis, as she had done so many times before. She nodded a greeting in my direction, acknowledging the initial management steps we'd taken, but the grimness in her eyes reflected our own. What was important now was to deliver the baby. Atsede and I knew what was coming, what was now necessary, and we already had everything prepared. Dr Rita confirmed what Atsede had found, or rather hadn't found, with an ultrasound of the baby's still, unmoving heart.

There are ways to manage such a situation, each with their own advantages and disadvantages. Sometimes, to wait is the least invasive course of action. But do you risk it? Waiting until the bones of the foetal skull soften and collapse inwards can finally release the baby and their mother from the ordeal that is a true obstructed labour. But to do so is playing with fire; wait too long and a hole may form as a result of the pressure on the soft, delicate tissue of the birth canal, leading to a chronic and devastating condition known as obstetric fistula, leaving women with a constant leaking of urine. No mention of fistula in Ethiopia can be made without a tribute to inspirational surgeon Dr Hamlin, a pioneer in low-resource fistula surgery and subsequent rehabilitation, who, until her sad passing at 96 years old in early 2020, was the matriarch of the Hamlin Fistula Hospital in Addis Ababa. The moving story of her and her husband's tireless work for women suffering from this appalling condition, as well as the challenges they faced, is laid bare in *The Hospital by the River*.

Along with the potential formation of a fistula, there is the shockingly high risk of infection for the mother from the slowly decomposing body of her stillborn child. Often, for women like Tsigey who are so unwell, relieving the extra pressure maintaining a pregnancy places on the body works miracles. Given that Tsigey had deteriorated further even in the short time since she'd arrived, would Dr Rita decide to take Tsigey to the operating theatre? Would that be better? To slice through the protective anatomy of the uterus to deliver the baby whose heartbeat and breath she'll never feel, whose hand she'll never hold. Would Tsigey thank us for that immediate kindness, given that in her next pregnancy she may not access midwifery or medical care, or fully comprehend the further, future risks to herself?

I am, for the second time that night, left wondering how you make a choice when there are no good options, and wondering about the toll on clinicians like Atsede and Dr Rita, who must, ultimately, make such decisions. The course of management left for Dr Rita for Tsigey was what is known as a craniotomy. It is a brutal, violent procedure that might just save her. Not many practitioners are able, or willing, to perform it safely. But here it was her only chance, and the only way. By perforating the foetal skull through mechanical enlargement of the fontanelle, tissue can be drained, reducing the circumference of the head, and, with clamps applied to the remaining cranial structures, a delivery can be facilitated. Although I try to think about it like this, in only technical terms, the horror of boring a hole into a baby's head to pull out their brain reduces me to tears every time. It still feels like an attack on the sanctity of the body, on the innocence of a child, on the love of a mother.

I'd assisted Dr Rita with the procedure before, determined not to shy away from any of the difficult realities of midwifery and obstetrics here, but no matter how many times nor for how many reasons it is necessary, I am always unprepared. The reality of life in rural Ethiopia is that the hospital often sees tough procedures and testing cases, from home circumcisions performed incorrectly to significant foetal abnormalities that have gone undetected, but the craniotomies are the only ones that still leave me rushing for the door, and taking long, deep breaths of cool air to recover. The moment I was no longer needed after Dr Rita had finished, I made my way quickly outside to sit with my head in my hands, shaking, bringing up the tea I'd just had.

Heaving a sigh of sadness and resignation, I got up and, trying to control the maelstrom of my emotions, splashed cold water on my face from the tap just outside the delivery room door. A glance up the avenue of huge, ancient trees that guarded the side of the hospital revealed that the first rays of pink and orange light were just finding their way through the clouds. Dawn was coming, bringing a new day.

Atsede, tougher and more stoic, glanced up as I entered, her eyes crinkling in sympathy, then went back to her vigil, sitting quietly with Tsigey, waiting for her to awaken, and I knew from the expression on her face and her barely moving lips that she was going over what she would say about what had happened. Before Tsigey came round, though, we had a few last things to do. Foremost among them was preparing the body of the baby for Tsigey or her relatives to take home if they wished. A little less than half of stillborn babies are laid to rest by their families, with most buried in a small graveyard behind the hospital. While it's a beautiful place, with swaying eucalyptus and bright red bottle-brush, the hyenas that prowl the perimeter fences have been known to disinter the graves if they are not dug deep enough.

There is little ceremony to the task of wrapping the baby, and although I'm not sure what I believe about what happens after death, each time it falls to me, I try to clarify my thoughts enough to send up a plea for the soul of the baby who never made it into the world. Something to mark their humanity, acknowledge their existence. Because stillborn babies aren't christened, there is no formal burial service among either the Christian or Muslim populations who make up the patients. And yet, I want the baby to find his way on, whatever and wherever that may mean. I had asked Atsede many months ago how she handled it. As a devout Catholic, she turns to prayer, and it's not unusual to find her eyes closed and hands clasped over a tiny body, lips moving silently, entrusting their fate to God. Whether Atsede's prayers, or my less specific but just as heartfelt requests for help, make any difference, we'll never know. But every life, no matter how fleeting, matters.

Wrapping a baby who has been through a craniotomy is not an easy thing. Much like after an autopsy, when the technicians try to remodel the empty body to something resembling normal, my shaking hands and shaking heart tried to tie bits of cut-off IV tubing in such a way that the collapsed skull would be less apparent. Knowing that the baby might be unwrapped once more, should Tsigey decide to take him home, I remembered at the last moment the stack of baby hats I had seen in one of the drawers in the linen cupboard earlier that day. Leaving a starched white cloth over the baby's body, I went quickly to find it, but on my return simply stood with it in my hands wondering what to do. The depth of poverty here means babies often have no clothes and no bonnets, no soft blankets or cotton swaddles, but are simply wrapped in old cloth. This hat could make a difference to another baby, to a living baby, for many days or weeks. It would only be buried with Tsigey's. And yet I found myself trying to work it on to what remained of the baby's skull. Atsede glanced in my direction, and my hands stilled, a pause in my attempts as I looked at her, with my eyes full of both tears and questions. For the longest moment she watched before half-raising a shoulder. She didn't have any more answers than I did. And so, with a beautiful, pale blue, hand-knitted hat covering our butchery, I finished wrapping Tsigey's baby, and whispered my entreaty and wish that things had been different, reflecting on the heavy burden that this young woman would now carry with her forever. Turning to my next task, cleaning the instruments, I heard stirrings behind the curtains. Tsigey was waking up. She was still very unwell, but the mere fact of her consciousness promised a chance at recovery. For her body, at least. Her mind and her heart might take far longer to heal.

Quickly, I went to find Kidist, and stood holding her hand tightly as Atsede explained what had happened. The tears streaked silently over Tsigey's cheeks as she turned her face away, unable, or unwilling, to look at any of us. Touching her shoulder lightly in expression of her sorrow and sympathy, Atsede moved away, motioning for me to join her, leaving Kidist and Tsigey to grieve together for what could, and should, have been.

Atsede

'Wait', came Indie's quiet voice, just as I reached out for the dented aluminium tin holding the instruments necessary for attending a birth. I paused, one hand on the lid, the other already encased in a sterile glove so held immobile, hovering in mid-air, away from anything that might contaminate it. My mind was on Melele, the beautiful woman lying on her side on the yellow plastic of the delivery trolley in front of me, whose baby it was my responsibility to bring into the world safely. But somewhere in my thoughts I noted for later that one corner of the tin was rusting. We would need another, newer one soon. And the box of gloves was running low, as were the used IV giving sets that we cut to fit into the end of a catheter and a used bag of IV fluids which acted as the collection reserve. The oxygen cylinders were empty too, I remembered. And in the morning, I would need to collect the money for the HIV women's peer support group. So many things to think about. 'Are you sure that's necessary?' Pulled back to the present, it took a moment to register Indie's hesitation.

I felt myself bristling, like the porcupine found among the *enset* trees in the garden, quills pulled upright and ready for a fight. I glanced over at Indie, standing just inside the pool of light cast by the wick of the candle lit to keep the darkness of night at bay. There was an earnest look in her eyes, but a weariness too. She rarely challenged my practice, understanding the experience and knowledge that working as a senior midwife in the hospital for almost a decade has given me. *Oh Indie,* I thought, *you're so caught up in being her advocate, you forget that I am on her side too.*

I'd tell Indie that, but later. Not now, when it was Melele we should be focused on. She had done well, so far, remaining calm and quiet, tracing a path around the room with slow steps, punctuated by pauses as she stilled, trying to breathe through the bunching of the powerful muscles of her uterus. She wasn't Gurage, but instead from the south, where the demons fly by night and magic rules. Her face, with cheekbones cast much higher and more prominently than ours tend to be, was marred only by an intricate arrangement of dots and lines; marking her family connections, she had told me earlier, when she could still make conversation. I had watched her walking on and off through the night, noting the spaces between the pauses growing closer, seeing her eyes cloud and close as the intensity of her contractions increased. For days and years, I had guided women through their labour, and knew the tell-tale signs of a birth coming closer. I motioned to the delivery trolley at the end, and pulled the curtains around us, creating our own little world, and started talking, saying nothing new really, just reassurances. She was nearly there, and I had just seen a flicker of the top of her baby's head when I heard Indie's footsteps padding quietly across the floor towards us. The caesarean had gone well then, if Indie was back so soon. I was pleased to have another set of hands to help, for one last time, to make sure Melele's blood pressure was staying within the normal limits. Her contractions were steady, her breathing was good, I could see her skin starting to stretch to make room for the passage of the baby's head. There were scars there too, just as intricately arranged as along her cheeks and over her forehead and chin, but far less by design. Like me, she had been circumcised. So while her skin would stretch, it was unlikely to be enough. I sighed, turning to open the delivery tin and ready the instruments needed to perform an episiotomy.

In a heartbeat, I can imagine the scene of her circumcision, coloured by the vague memories of my own but also those I had been aware of as part of the background tapestry of village life. In the midst of the green *enset* trees, with the loamy smells of rich, damp leaf mould, and the incessant chattering of the bright blue and red birds flitting through the fruit trees, the women would gather together. Some came with a young girl at their side, with their hands nervously wrapped in the long, colourful dresses of their mothers, whispering and giggling quietly with their friends. Behind the thatched kitchen, a circle of wood, a slice from a large tree, worn smooth by years of processing the roots of the *enset* to become the dough for *wussa*. Braced against it, the old woman with her wrinkled, solemn face from the ritually ambiguous Fugah tribe whose work it is to perform the circumcisions, along with shaping and firing the black clay *kawa jebena*, coffee pots, and serving dishes, *bitr,* ubiquitous in Gurage households.

The world would continue around this small group, gathered in the garden, with tight smiles on the faces of the women and vague apprehension in the eyes of the girls, not entirely sure what was to come. Early in the afternoon, before the sun reached its highest point and while there was still a breeze rustling through the branches heavy with avocado, mango, guava, or bananas, the zebu cows would be on their way to the village from the pastures, but the men who bring them would stay out of sight a little longer than normal, waiting before calling to their wives and daughters for small cups of hot, strong *kawa* and a plate heaped with fresh cheese or the spicy, lentil *wot*. The girls knew something was happening: they had seen the quiet preparations over the days gone by, the gathering of food, the *sahrbet* huts scrubbed with even more vigour than usual, the firewood stacked high in the corner. They had seen this before, with older sisters or cousins or aunts. They felt the excitement in the air. They knew something happened near the big block of wood, and that it made the older girls, the ones they so looked up to and admired, cry out, but then there was music and singing and dancing and food, and the night went on forever as the families celebrated.

The festivities continued until, at last, tired and joyful, the adults collapsed onto straw mats, wrapped in blankets, and slept. For the days afterwards, the older girls stayed inside, didn't have to help with washing clothes or sweeping the floors, and instead ate all the foods usually kept only for the big holidays, dark green kale cooked with rich butter and spices, fresh cheese, and even meat, finely diced and served raw as *kutfo*. There would be visitors, too, with women arriving carrying baskets of fruit or *injera*, brightly-coloured scarves twisted around their hair, and feet red from the dust still on the ground waiting for the *keremt* rains. The men would gather outside, sitting on the carved wooden stools, hands clasped across their chests or on the long, thick sticks resting on their knees, but the girls weren't as interested in them, given that they only sat and talked, drinking *kawa* during the day and shots of home-brewed, eye-watering *arakay* at night. It was the women who brought the gossip and the fruit and the laughter, who had time for the flock of girls trying to make away with bits of food before they were really supposed to, and who could even be persuaded into handing over a dented kettle and a handful of sugar so they could make sweet, wild mint tea with *nahnah* leaves foraged from the garden. They knew there was now a special tree in the garden, where a small package, wrapped in *enset ketel*, had been left high in the heart of the huge spreading leaves, imbibing some magical properties that would now allow the tree to produce the sweetest and most delicious *wussa*. When they asked, the women had chided their endless curiosities, and said simply that was what had been cut away. Shrugging, without fully understanding the implications, but satisfied that at least they had an answer of sorts, the girls ran off again, tumbling like kid goats, their imagination already caught up in the next mystery needing solving.

The same scenes played out every year, and now it was the tumbling girls' turn, my turn. With my hair neatly braided by my older sister, matching my cousin, Hana, who stood so close I could smell the sticky mango juice still drying on her hands, mingled with the smoke and the roasting *kawa*, I shifted my weight from one bare foot to the other, waiting. I surreptitiously rubbed my thigh, where it still stung from the slap my older sister had given me when I couldn't sit still as she had been getting me ready. More than the stinging, though, I could feel the kiss on my cheek that she'd given me when she was through, and hear her pronouncement that I was the most beautiful little rascal in all the world. Trying to peer ahead and see what was happening, I saw a smiling face appear between the tree trunks and stuck my tongue out at my younger brother and his rambunctious playmates, all of whom would soon be chased off by a harried older woman brandishing a length of sugar cane. Turning to Hana, giggling silently, I saw her eyes suddenly widen. Without us realising, too distracted by tracing the light footsteps of the boys through the garden as they ran away shouting and laughing, we had come to the front of the group of women. It was our turn to take our place sitting on the *zigba* wood.

I cannot remember the details exactly. I do remember feeling surprised, feeling the sharp pain of the razor blade, and the even sharper sting of a liquid sloshed on afterwards. It hurt beyond what I had expected, and the strength of the women holding me down frightened me as much as the glitter of the blade catching the sunlight. The passing thoughts of why my sisters and aunts and mother had allowed me to suffer like this, and then Hana crying out as she sat down after me, and wanting to hold her hand and tell her it was okay. And then the burning ache, for days, especially after having to pass water. But also the special food, the *kutfo*, and being able to stay without having to help around the house and garden, for seven days. But the specifics have faded, joining the other trials of a wild childhood spent in the trees and the river, where the cuts and scrapes and burns and bruises all left their mark. There were other injuries: none so deliberate, but my cousins had also had to hold me down while my aunt cleaned out a deep wound in my leg one day, a souvenir of playing on the stack of wood. And that too had been stitched up without anaesthesia.

These recollections of my circumcision played out in the endless seconds of Indie's question before more recent experiences flooded in and chased them out. These were of the women who had delivered at home without midwives, whose torn and ragged flesh was never properly repaired, and who suffered the searing pain of subsequent infections; of the women who succumbed after those same infections took hold and spread like wildfire through their bodies, destroying everything in their path, of the delirious staring and sweet, rotting scent of their dying bodies. I couldn't find the words to tell Indie though.

Instead, I felt a wave of sadness wash over me as I pictured the research sites she now spoke of. Looking around the delivery room I had carefully held together for so long, I wondered what it must be like to practise somewhere with reliable electricity, a constant, clean water supply, the ability to simply write down any drug or piece of equipment and know it would be available before too long. I had read those papers too. And looked at the names of the authors and hospitals where the studies were undertaken. They certainly weren't Gurage, nor even Ethiopian or Kenyan,

Somalian, Sudanese, or Ugandan. They weren't the names of women and midwives who had births like we did. The hospital, run as it is by missionary nuns, had seen a handful of visiting midwives over the years. Many had tried to insist that episiotomies weren't necessary, using the same evidence. Many had then had to call me over to repair the difficult, complex consequences of their actions. But these were consequences that played out on another woman's body, not their own. Their black and white theory failing to adhere to the shades of grey of life. They didn't understand, and weren't willing to listen, with an unshakeable belief in their degrees and their certificates. I respected and adored Indie though, and knew she felt the same about me, so I thought she would listen.

We had spoken about circumcision before, and it was through those conversations that I had marshalled my amorphous and conflicting feelings on it into formative words and sentences. Without circumcision, there was the fear that girls would become wilful, argumentative, and headstrong, none of which were desirable in a place and a time where women were expected to be complacent and docile, minding the words and wants first of their fathers and brothers, and later their husbands. This discourse runs deep, to the heart of our language, and even now, there is no insult as hurtful as *ohfoh*, the word used to describe an uncircumcised woman. I believe that we were not cut as girls to cause pain and difficulty, but instead because it was the given thing to do, and there was the pervasive understanding that it would help us to learn to control our sexual selves, the part of us also responsible for such unbecoming behaviour as disobedience. In a way, having now studied the biology and anatomy that lies behind the practice, I have to concede that this is, in many ways, an effective, albeit cruel, means of achieving that. Once the parts of our body that allow us to feel that particular pleasure are cut off, and hidden away in the branches of the *enset*, why would we seek out men to take to a darkened corner? In many ways, we are lucky. Our circumcision is not as brutal as elsewhere. Unlike the tall, dark women in their billowing blue or black robes from Somalia and northern Kenya, where just their eyes, outlined in kohl, are visible, the alterations to our Gurage bodies are far less marked. And yet still enough to cause pain, still enough to cause problems in childbirth, still enough.

Knowing what Melele was facing, I sent a silent, grateful thanks to my mother, and my village, that my sister would never experience this. I was among the last to be circumcised, with the practice starting to fade just a handful of years later. I hold no resentment, or anger, towards the women in my family. I understand that they were acting in what they believed to be my best interest, and simply had never been given reason to question it. I understand they simply carried forth the ideas of the women that walked before them. I understand they acted out of love, not malice, because they thought it was necessary for upholding honour and purity. I understand. But I also know that the practice had to stop. I know that the complications and traumas and difficulties faced by girls who are circumcised are not necessary, and more, are not constructive. I know women's bodies do not need to be altered in order to be more acceptable to men. I know that circumcision isn't a religious requirement, not written of in the Bible or the Qu'ran, and I know that God would not create women as so imperfect that parts of our bodies needed removing. So I understand, but I know better. And this, really, is the key to seeing circumcision stop entirely. In the knowing. It is this that enables the strong pull of culture to be cast aside. So many programmes and eradication campaigns start from the premise that they are working against us, that we will staunchly defend our practices, against all reason. But this isn't true. With patience, and education, and understanding, the older women (for raising children here is the realm of women, not men) can, and will, see through the fog of their cultural bias and realise that it isn't in the best interest of their girls. And the men will see the difficulties, and stand up, and say that it must not be done in their name. With that, circumcision will stop. It happened in my village. It will happen elsewhere too. There's an ancient Amharic proverb that translates to something like 'from milk, butter can be made'. It means that with patience and perseverance, great things can be achieved, even if they take a little time. Changing traditions and cultures is like that.

Indie and I had been sitting with a friend of ours, Askalech, one afternoon in the Clinic. She'd come for antenatal care, and an ultrasound scan of the tiny new life that had just started to move around enough to be felt. It was such a hot day that we had done everything we needed inside quickly, then retreated to the breeze of the veranda, where we could sit on the cool tiles and lean against the cool walls. Part of the conversations we have are around what to expect during the birth itself. I asked Askalech about her circumcision, knowing she is Hadiya, where more severe forms are sometimes seen. She explained that she didn't think hers was severe, as she had no problems passing her water or at night with her husband. As she told us about her experience, though, explaining that she had been circumcised in a hospital, by a nurse, using sterile instruments, with local anaesthesia, and given prophylactic antibiotics and analgesia to take away, I could see Indie's, and feel my own, disbelief mounting. This was what I had read about. The medicalisation of circumcision. Askalech had no way of knowing that this information would be of any particular interest to us, so she had no reason to make it up. I flinched knowing that midwives and nurses, trained as I was, to the same clinical standards, were willing to perform such procedures. Then faint recollections of another conversation surfaced in my mind. It was with a nurse who had come wanting an HIV test after sustaining a needlestick injury, an occupational hazard for healthcare professionals the world over. Indie had been seeing to her, and, trying to keep the conversation light and reassuring, had been teasing her about what she must have been doing for this to happen. Almost without realising, the nurse had replied that she was doing circumcisions. And she had used the nuance to the word that suggested this was female, not male, which is also customary here. The subtleties of Amharic tend to pass Indie by, but I had picked up on it, and asked her more. Several minutes later, it came out that she was, to all intents and purposes, a cutter. The shock must have shown on both of our faces, because she was quick to justify her actions. If she performed 'circumcision' in the hospital, with local anaesthesia, then all she had to do was spend enough time going through the motions of a procedure, and draw a little blood to put on a white gauze and look impressive, and the family would be content. Comprehension spread across Indie's face, mirrored, I was certain, on my own. The nurse had been educated in the complications, and understood the implications, of what circumcising women means, and so, to protect girls from the butchery of the village circumcisers, she put on a charade. It was a brave operation. Were she to be found out, not only would she face the legal ramifications of getting caught up in a practice illegal in Ethiopia, but she would also face the wrath of the families of the girls she had seen over the years. Indie found it harder to come to terms with than I did, but even she understood the risks the nurse was taking to look out for the girls.

Breaking through my reverie was the low groan of a coming contraction, and the swell of Melele's stomach rising up underneath my hand; with it my focus shifted back to the present. Glancing at the watch hanging from Indie's scrub top pocket, I filled in the details of what I was feeling. Still on her side, Melele had one hand slung up over her head, her fingers dangling, moving to the rhythm of her breathing, and the other hand tight around the drip stand holding the curtain away from the bed. Again, the groan, and more of the top of a dark head of hair becoming visible. Along with it, the tightness of skin unable to stretch.

'Forgive me', I whisper, as much to myself, and to women across Ethiopia whose circumcision necessitates this, as to Melele, before explaining a little louder what I thought needed to happen now. Tears sprang to her eyes, but she nodded, determined. With the start of the next contraction, and with Melele's concentration turned inward, I had the scissors in place. Wincing at the pain I knew was coming for her, not just now but in the days and weeks after, I held my breath as Indie held her tongue, and made a quick, sharp cut. In the next instant, with a gush of warm, clear fluid, Melele's daughter is born. She's quiet, but her eyes open softly as I place her close to her mother's breast, and lift Melele's tired hand to cover her back. Her fists clench and release, one leg stretching out, and she tries to blink the amniotic waters out of her eyes. A tiny sneeze. The minutes pass as Melele and her daughter lie there, oblivious to the world around them, caught up in getting to know each other, and Indie and I stand quietly by, waiting for the telltale signs of the separation of her placenta. We watched as the umbilical cord faded to white, and I eased it out from underneath the warm little body, motioning to Indie for the clamps. Melele's daughter, for better or worse, was her own, separate entity. And although she would still rely on Melele for everything, in her arms rather than her belly, it was the first step to independence.

It was a small blessing for Melele that the wards were quiet tonight, that we didn't have ten other women close to delivery. It isn't unusual for us here to be running between beds, with just enough time to scrub our hands and change gloves between catching baby after baby. The unhurried atmosphere, the candlelight, the cool darkness of night, lent a timelessness to the moment. Melele took her time touching her baby's fine eyebrows, tracing her hairline, stroking her cheek. It was only when I came out of the shadows where I had been sitting and writing her notes, to ask if I could repair the damage I had inflicted with my scissors, that Melele noticed we were there at all. She gritted her teeth, grimacing at the sharp bite of the needle with eyes clenched shut. But when her baby voiced her first cry, hungry no doubt, Melele's concentration snapped to her instead. Within minutes, I had repaired the episiotomy site. Happy with how her muscles and skin had come back together, I quietly reminded Melele of the importance of trying to stay clean, of using fresh cloth in her underwear, and only boiled water to wash herself. I offered to help dress the baby, and as Indie moved around unobtrusively in the background, gathering the instruments for cleaning and the blood-stained clothes for laundering, I found the plastic carrier bag Melele had stashed under the bed in the postnatal room she had chosen as her own all those hours ago when she first arrived. In it was a long, colourful kaftan, the unofficial uniform of women here, and a tshirt for the baby. With an old, folded towel as her nappy, I watched as she deftly wrapped the baby in a blanket and placed her in the waiting arm of her sister, then offered to help Melele to the bathing room. Indie had already carried in two buckets of warm water, the small wooden stool, and a bar of soap.

Clean, warm, and dressed in her fresh clothes, Melele wandered back to the resting room and lay down, smiling, on the starched white sheet pulled over the bright yellow mattress. Her daughter at her breast, and her sister by her side, she closed her eyes and slept.

Standing, leaning against the doorframe, watching Melele, I heard the clink of metal, and the slosh of water being stirred up with soap granules. Turning, I saw that Indie had started washing the instruments, and remembered our disagreement, not liking the friction between us. I sighed, and walked across to join her, putting on gloves and holding a hand out for one of the toothbrushes used to clean the inner blades of the scissors and clamps.

'Will you tell me about it?' It was Indie's voice, and I could hear the apology in it, the interest too. She genuinely wanted to know; she wasn't just asking because she thought she ought to. I felt myself smiling, and turned to her, ready for the conversation.

We were still talking about the cases I'd seen, the repairs I'd had to redo, and the ones I couldn't, when Indie took the bucket of hot, soapy water to scrub down the bed space. I was explaining the depth of the complexity. It wasn't as simple as worrying about the tearing. Afterwards, when these women go home, they often just don't have the ability to keep wounds, especially those that extend beyond the muscles of the perineum and instead reach into the muscles further down and around, that control the anal sphincter, as clean as needed to promote proper healing. Water is often scarce, carried to the house on the backs of the women in yellow jerrycans. Indie nodded, grinning ruefully, no doubt thinking of the times she and I had done just this, with me laughing at her attempts to hoist the heavy, dripping cans off her back without soaking everything in sight. Mattresses, sheets, clothes, underwear: while the women try their best, keeping these clean is difficult in a land of dust and smoke and cattle. What's more, without comprehensive community-based midwifery, clinical postnatal care is limited. So even if women are starting to wonder if their wounds aren't healing properly, it would take them travelling to a health facility to get any sort of assessment. This isn't easy with a newborn, a painful wound, only public transport, and often half an hour or more of walking, either in hot sunshine or heavy rain. I spoke on and on, needing Indie to understand the complexities and challenges that Gurage women just like me face, how the health inequalities are compounded by the circumstances of poverty. The Gurage lands are beautiful, but difficult.

I could see that Indie was beginning to understand, but was still grappling with the magnitude of the choices clinicians here have to make. After thousands of hours and thousands of births, I now accept the responsibilities I have as the midwife. It is in my hands and my heart where the heavy weight of life and death rest. If I think about it too much, it takes my breath away, but then the next woman walks in, and I'm ready to make the decisions once more. Indie's attention is suddenly caught by something, and I see her head come up at the same time I hear the rattling wheels of a trolley careening down the corridor in haste. Time to go.

'What is it? What's going on?' I looked into the worried eyes of Meka, the nurse from the Emergency Room. He spoke in hurried, frantic tones, reading from the slip of a referral paper, eyes constantly darting back to the patient on the trolley, clearly worried about her condition. With one glance, I could see why. Her eyes, bruised blue from tiredness, were closed, her head lolled to one side, the rise and fall of her chest barely discernible. Talking quickly with the young woman at her side, who stood clutching a plastic bag in her arms and a small, folded square of paper in her hand, which she held out helplessly, I ran through in my mind what we were to do now. Reaching over Tsigey, the name of the girl lying silent on the trolley, I felt in the drawer for the pinard and, lifting up her sodden dress, held it to her abdomen. I didn't expect to hear anything, not after she had laboured for three endless days, but was saddened by the silence nonetheless. Obstructed labour is one of the most torturous emergencies for women to experience. They are healthy, their baby is well, their pregnancy is simple, their labour even starts normally. And then it simply doesn't stop. The labour goes on and on, and without intervention, there is no hope for the child. Often a stillbirth, at times a fistula, rupture, bleeding, sepsis. In that sense, Tsigey is lucky. Her sister, the woman with the plastic bag, insisted she be brought to hospital. Here, at least, we can try and save her.

'Get everything ready, Indie. I'll go to Dr Rita.' Pausing only to throw a blanket over my shoulders against the cold, I made my way quickly out of the door and across the crunching stones to the gates at the end of the road. There, I knocked on the glass window of the guard house, rousing Tigistu from his reverie. A small bonfire was burning just outside, and he had a steaming mug of *kawa* between his hands. I smiled a quick greeting before Tigistu stood up, stretched, and walked quickly to knock on the door of a sleeping Dr Rita. A few minutes later he was back, with the scraping of a key in the lock and the clanging of the big metal gates swinging open.

'Good morning, Atsede. What have you got for me?' Dr Rita, the unflappable Medical Director of the hospital, who had given her life to the women here. As we marched back up the road, her white coat still over her arms as she cleaned her glasses, I took Dr Rita through Tsigey's story. We reached the ward, and I led the way back in through the sluice side door, Dr Rita following a heartbeat later. She was at Tsigey's side in a few strides, taking in the IV, the oxygen, the catheter, nodding in appreciation of the treatment we had initiated. As Dr Rita checked Tsigey over, I wheeled the old ultrasound machine across to her, Indie handing me a bottle of the thick blue gel as I went. With the confirmation of intrauterine death, Dr Rita stepped back, shook her head with heaviness, and asked for the craniotomy set. I had suspected this would happen, so already had it open and waiting on one of the wheeled stainless-steel tables. As the senior midwife, I always had to be available to respond to the changing needs of the ward, which meant it fell on Indie to assist Dr Rita. I knew how she felt about craniotomies, but I also knew she was learning to come to terms with the unkindness of an act designed only to save the life of the mother. The one good thing that can be said about the procedure is that Dr Rita is able to complete it quickly. As I monitored the postnatal women, and admitted several antenatal women, my mind was on the closed curtains, and on Tsigey's sister, sitting on the floor outside, staring silently at the floor, occasionally heaving a shaking sigh. I wanted to go to her, offer words of reassurance, but until I knew that Tsigey would be okay, giving false hope would be worse than the silence. With the tell-tale squeak of the door leading outside opening, I knew it was over, and that would be Indie, giving in to her sadness in the dawn air. Quickly finishing the restocking of gloves, and labelling the empty oxygen cylinders, I caught up with Dr Rita just as she was peeling her gloves off and standing to leave. 'You'll need a new delivery set tin soon, Atsede, that one is rusting around the corners. Remind me in the morning.' She missed nothing. The craniotomy had been a success, in so much as that the baby was delivered, and there was no further damage to Tsigey. Little would that lessen the pain of telling her what had happened. I nodded my thanks, and bade Dr Rita goodnight as she headed home for a few more hours sleep before getting up to run the hospital. I turned a circle, looking for one of the chairs to pull up beside Tsigey, and tried to work out how to say what I needed to. Her vital signs had stabilised in the quarter of an hour or so since her baby had been delivered, and the fluids had started to rehydrate her after the hours and hours of fruitless labouring. The door squeaked once more, and I opened the curtain a little to see Indie walking in, pale but determined. I caught her eye, but my mind was still on what to say.

The next time I glanced up, now with a script in mind for Tsigey once she woke, it was to find Indie standing, staring at the knitted hat in her hand. In a moment, I understood exactly the turmoil of her thoughts; should she use this hat for Tsigey's baby, given it would likely be buried in a handful of hours, or should she put it down, and wait for another, live baby who would benefit far more from its warmth? This was Indie's decision, and I had no answer for her, so just raised a shoulder in response to the question in her eyes. She must do what she believes to be best. I watched as she tried to get the hat to stay on, and when at last she succeeded, she paused for a moment. I knew she was praying for the soul of the baby; I had seen it many times. Stillbirths and neonatal deaths are an inescapable part of midwifery. There is nothing as sad as visiting a friend or relative, curled on their side on the bed, an empty space next to them where their baby should be, with aching breasts and an aching heart. Here, these women are still referred to using the same language as those with a living baby, they are still treated as new mothers, they still thought of as having a child, just in a different place. Visitors come, bringing sweet mango juice or *kawa* beans. They stay a few minutes, the men outside the bedroom but still in earshot, the women sitting on low stools beside her bed, to hear her story. She will talk to each one, and each time she speaks of what happened it gets a little easier to bear. Without fail, there will be long minutes spent with every member of her family, her friends, her neighbours, and for three months she will be surrounded by love and sympathy and sadness, able to rest and grieve, with meals brought for her and all her household tasks seen to. And, somehow, eventually, it will help her to heal. In a land where so many women have lost babies, there is a tacit understanding that in walking this sad path, you are not alone. Tsigey, too, will join the women before her who have been through this. She will join two of my sisters, my mother, my aunt, several friends. Inevitably women from her own life. As I think about this, I feel rather than see a shift in the air around her. She is waking up. As Tsigey starts to move, Indie notices and quickly makes her way out, to bring Kidist, I'm sure. They come back through the door not long after, in time to see Tsigey blink heavily and start to lift her head from the pillow. I talk in low tones, pausing often to give the sisters a chance to take on board what I am saying, and explain what happened. At some point, Tsigey starts to weep silently, the tears tracing across her cheeks and pooling on her scarf. Kidist's eyes fill too, but in hers it is possible also to see overwhelming relief. She witnessed Tsigey's deterioration and collapse, and even after she had handed her sister to us, she wasn't sure if she would ever see her alive again. I reach out, gently resting my fingers on her shoulder, wanting Tsigey to understand that I am sorry that this has happened to her, that she will never see her baby grow up, that she will miss him forever. I know my words won't provide comfort, not really; it is the warmth and care of those closest to her she needs now. As Kidist steps forward, I step away, and motion to Indie to join me. We left them together, Kidist's arms wrapped around her little sister protectively, giving her the space and time to start her mourning, and start her healing.

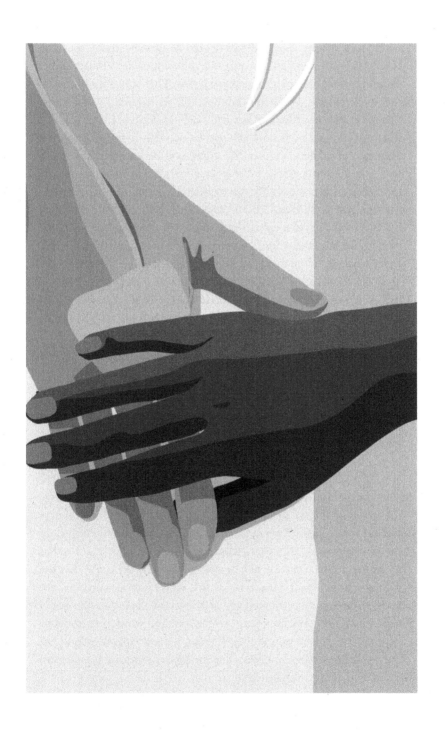

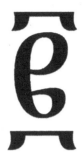

2

Tizazu

Indie

I tried, again, to explain why it mattered. 'But everyone is someone's child', I say, beseeching, imploring Atsede to give in, to understand. When I give blood to women who have lost too much during a birth, I can usually put a stop to her objections by simply saying, 'one day, it could be you'. It is an area of our beliefs that, unusually, sees us standing in stark opposition to one another. I believe that anyone able to give blood is morally bound to do so. I'm yet to work out to whom, or what, they are bound; perhaps to the concept of the sanctity of life, or God or Allah if that is their highest authority, but that doesn't detract from the imperative. More than that, if you would be willing to accept blood for yourself or your family, then how can you not also be willing to give it? Atsede, on the other hand, doesn't think this, and neither of us are willing to concede an inch. With blood that can be given to anybody – a universal donor as it's known – I'm often called on in emergencies. Dr Rita knows I have no blood-borne diseases, and that I am, thankfully, healthy and willing. She lies me down, places a big bore cannula in the crook of my elbow, and fills a special bag sent from Germany with my blood. Still warm, the bag is then taken to where it is needed, often with me following a few minutes later, and the transfusion can start. The impact of fresh, whole blood cannot be understated, and even when all seems lost, women on the brink come back. The tell-tale plaster over the donation site receives raised eyebrows from Atsede every time, but she knows me well enough to not argue. It is the simplest, most straightforward way for any one person to directly contribute towards saving another person's life, not just in Ethiopia, but across the world, and yet still, somehow, there are shortages every day in every country.

We were sitting, now, side-by-side on the bench outside the long, low building that temporarily housed the Neonatal Unit, looking in through the windows at the woman sitting at the cotside of a baby earlier diagnosed with a subdural haematoma. He was stable, for now, but the morning's blood sample I'd collected and walked to the lab had come back showing a worryingly low haemoglobin level and a rising white cell count. I was nervous. I watched the baby twitching in his sleep, his little belly rounded out after a breastfeed, and then settle under his mother's loving caresses. He was a sweet looking thing, with his black hair already tightly curled and fine eyebrows arching above big, dark eyes. He was pale though, a common result of anaemia, and his heartbeat, when I checked for his half-hourly observations, was far too fast. I didn't want him to deteriorate even further, to a place from where we couldn't bring him back. I'd tracked down Atsede and Selam, and brought them here to help me with a treatment plan, but Atsede, at least, was resistant. To correct his plummeting haemoglobin levels, a blood transfusion was the best way forward. But blood here is difficult to come by. The hospital often runs out, and relatives are hesitant to donate their own, even when their loved one's life depends on it.

Atsede protested because it was only days before that I'd given blood to a woman suffering the effects of a placental abruption that had already claimed the life of her thirdborn, and which, without blood, would soon have taken hers too. Because of how limited the blood supplies are, willing donors among the hospital staff are not called upon for women who will probably die, only for those who will probably survive, as each can only give so much at one time, and it is better to save it for those who stand a chance. It doesn't always work out like that though. Each time we get it wrong, and I sit at the dinner table with the nuns who run the hospital with resignation in my voice, Sister Inge offers soft words of commiseration that always include the idea that part of me went with her to heaven. While I like the thought, and take some comfort from it, I fervently wish, every time, that it wasn't the case.

It was because I truly believed that if we intervened now we could save Tizazu before it was too late, that I was still arguing my case with Atsede. As fate would have it, the baby's blood type was the same as mine, reducing his chances of finding another willing donor to next to nothing. Atsede stood by her objection, adamant that I shouldn't jeopardise my own health by donating again so soon. Knowing this would be her concern, I offered the rationalisation for my plan: this transfusion would require far less from me, and I could just take it easy over the next week or so, and eat well. I would recover, but without blood the baby might not. 'And what if there's another woman tomorrow?' Atsede said, just as certain she was right, just as unwilling to concede an inch. 'You know how often we see emergencies; it could happen. When do you say enough is enough?'. We both looked to Selam, wanting her to weigh in with an opinion that would break the deadlock. She looked back, preoccupied with the fate of the baby, but grinned on seeing our identical expressions of exasperated earnestness as Atsede and I both implored her to get on our side.

'Atsede, Indie is right...' Selam started to say.

'Yes! Thank yo- '

'I haven't finished. Indie is right that a blood transfusion is the best course of action. But Indie, Atsede is right in that you are only human, you have a finite amount of blood that you need to keep you healthy. You can't just keep draining it out. You'll not be able to help anyone if you become unwell.'

A little chagrined, I was nevertheless touched by their concern. And in my heart of hearts I knew that they were right. But I needed them to be right another day with another patient. Not today, with this one. A compromise, then. Slinging an arm over each of their shoulders, and planting a kiss on each of their cheeks, I used my most cajoling voice, promising that I absolutely and definitely wouldn't so much as give a drop for the next three months if I could just help this baby now. As Atsede clenched her teeth to stop from smiling, glancing at Selam with comical despair, I knew I had won. So, the preparations began.

Selam, as well as being an experienced midwife, had spent many shifts on the high dependency children's ward, so we decided she would manage Tizazu, while I would be in Atsede's capable hands. Tizazu needed weighing, how much blood was required needed calculating, and we both needed cannulas sited. But we couldn't go ahead with such a procedure unless we had the agreement of Dr Rita, and it was up to me to present the case and proposed treatment to her. I gathered the notes, the most recent lab results, and my courage, and made my way through the hospital to the gynaecological outpatients' room, where I'd heard it on good authority that Dr Rita was screening women for cervical cancer. With a distracted wave to enter as I pulled back the screen, as promised I found Dr Rita writing up the notes from her last patient. I smiled with apprehension and perched on the edge of the bed, spreading the papers in front of us, and then, with a deep breath, I began. I explained about the traumatic delivery, about the baby's growing head circumference, the falling haemoglobin, the hope in the eyes of his mother when I said I had a plan, the tentative agreement of Atsede and Selam in helping. I watched as concern, scepticism, and then comprehension flitted across her face, along with something that seemed akin to pride, which touched and emboldened me in equal measure. We had a good team, and we had a good plan. Could we go ahead? The wait while Dr Rita went meticulously through every detail, especially our calculations as to how much blood was enough, seemed to go on for ever. And then, as simply as that, she signed the treatment form. A wave of relief washed over me with the flush of victory – we could go ahead. And more than that, Dr Rita would come and assist. It isn't often that direct donor-recipient blood transfusions happen in the hospital, particularly with a baby, and she wanted to make sure everything went according to plan.

Without the certainties of a blood banking system, the transfusions themselves would have to be quick. The blood couldn't be allowed to clot. Not in my cannula, the syringes, or Tizazu's. For it to do so would be very dangerous. Atsede, Selam, and I, as part of the preparation, had spent an hour reading about direct blood transfusions. Although arterial to venous, from an artery in my arm to one of the veins in Tizazu's, used to be how such transfusions were done decades ago, the control of the speed of transfusion, and the amount transfused, was far more difficult, and with a system as delicate as that of baby just a few days old, the margins of error were small, and risks of getting it wrong were too high. The best option, it seemed, would be venous to venous, with a syringe bridging the gap. This would be a dance of sorts, with Atsede taking enough from me to fill a syringe that would be given to Tizazu quickly enough that the blood didn't clot but not so quickly that it ruptured his veins. Selam, nervous about the details and determined to honour her role as Tizazu's nurse and protect her charge, insisted we found a way to work that detail out before we went ahead. How peculiar it would have seemed to anyone looking in the window, with the three of us hunched over a white clothed cardboard box in front of syringes of various sizes filled with tiny amounts of my blood, with a clock propped up behind them counting the seconds until it coagulated and could only be pushed out with some force.

With the trial run finished, now certain we knew what to do, and with Dr Rita standing quietly in the corner watching over us, I took my seat at the cotside as Atsede and Selam prepared the cannulation kits and syringes, and scrubbed up. Staying scrupulously sterile was also a key factor; the last thing we wanted was to push potentially contaminated cells into Tizazu's blood and body.

Now we had started, there was an air of expectant hope in the air. We could do this. With a last raised eyebrow in my direction, reflecting the grin I knew was hidden under the blue paper face mask, Atsede motioned for my arm, where the tourniquet was already applied, trapping my blood in my veins and raising them up, making it easier for her to find one. The sting of a wide-bore needle finding the right place, and Tizazu's angry cry indicating it was the same for him, and we were ready. Dr Rita led, telling Atsede when to draw up, and Selam how fast to push it through.

For all our preparation, the transfusion itself was over in a matter of minutes. Now, there was nothing to do but wait. Tizazu's cannula was out, and he was nestled in the crook of his mother's arm, taking comfort in her closeness and her milk. Over the next few days we would watch his progress, expecting his anaemia to improve, his haematoma to stabilise and settle, and his tiny body to start to recover.

As the days passed by, it seemed the transfusion, the medication regime, and our whispered pleas had worked. Tizazu went from strength to strength, delighting his mother with gurgles and coos, and delighting us with falling infection markers and rising haemoglobin. Inevitably, between caring for women on the Delivery Suite and children on the Paediatric Ward, Selam, Atsede and I would drift back to our hard, wooden benches outside the Neonatal Unit, poring over his latest test results with smiles of relief. Atsede, in particular, knew what it meant to me for Tizazu to recover. The last few weeks had been difficult, and we were both still reeling from a case with an outcome far sadder than Tizazu's.

Birabiro had come from far away, birthed at home with little warning. His mother was young, and he was her first child. Now accustomed to the simple fact that limited antenatal care often means that babies with congenital conditions go undiagnosed, I wasn't too concerned when the phone call came saying that a new baby 'with something wrong' needed admitting to the Neonatal Unit. It was late in the day, the air thick and heavy with the rain that would come that evening. For the last few days the Unit had been nearly empty, an unusual lull that I didn't like, my midwife's intuition prickling uncomfortably. The three babies that I did have were thankfully stable, their daily routines no longer disturbed by hourly vital sign checks. Two out of three were breastfeeding without issue, and the vivacious, laughing mother of the third was having little problem expressing and syringe-feeding her tiny son, delivered early by caesarean section after her blood pressure rose beyond our means to control it, her hands and feet swollen with the tell-tale sign of severe pre-eclampsia. Zewdu was much recovered now she had her son safe in her arms, and kept us all giggling with her animated tales of the cow that fell into her long drop, and the chickens that will not leave her harassed cat alone. It's a challenging time, with a baby too sick or too small to safely take home, but having women like Zewdu there, keeping everyone smiling and taking them away, if only for the duration of her latest story, from their worries for their beloved child, is a medicine far beyond anything the staff can prescribe. I found myself grinning with anticipation as I walked along the red-tiled veranda, wondering what she would be regaling us with during the evening medication rounds, my vague trepidation over the new admission all but forgotten.

Stepping through the swinging door of the Unit, though, I was struck by the silence. The chatter of the three women lying in beds perpendicular to each other, passing *kawa* and roasted barley between them, that provided the normal soundtrack to the Neonatal Unit was non-existent. Even the babies were quiet, and it was as if the heaviness of the air outside had somehow amplified in here. A juddering sigh punctuated the stillness, and, frowning, I looked to its source. Huddled around the low bed on the ground just inside the door were two women, in the arms of one a bundle of cloth that, I could only assume, held the baby in question. Surreptitiously, I glanced at Zewdu. Her natural leadership and approachable nature had led her to be the unofficial spokeswoman for the Unit, and I had come to rely on her ability to quickly identify any struggling women and let me know what we could do to help. But, unusually, she wouldn't meet my eye, looking down instead at her hands on her lap, where they were fiddling with a loose thread. Feeling decidedly nervous, I glanced back out of the doors I had just come through, relieved to see one of the nurses from the Laboratory taking a sheaf of blood test results back to the Delivery Room. I caught his attention, and mouthed to him to get Atsede, please. I needed her reassuring presence.

Turning back to the silence of the room, I introduced myself to the two women, explaining that I was one of the clinicians in charge of the Neonatal Unit, and that we were here to look after babies who needed a little more help than usual. At those words, tears fell thickly from the downcast eyes of the younger woman, soaking her hijab. She looked exhausted, and desperately sad. The older woman – her mother, I wondered – started to answer the basic questions I was asking, how old the baby was, when they were born, how many months they thought the pregnancy lasted, stalling for time before Atsede arrived. Moments later came the creaking swing of the door, and I turned to see not only Atsede but also Dula, the gentlest, kindest man I've known, and the most compassionate nurse. Relief washed over me, and I sent a silent thanks to the laboratory nurse for his foresight in sending Dula too. Atsede nodded for me to continue, while Dula stepped up beside me, motioning for the younger woman to hand over the bundle. The act of passing your child into the hands, and trust, of another human is so simple, and yet so fraught, so difficult, so complicated. Her reluctance was clear, and it was as if her hands were bound to the child as tightly as her heart was.

Softly, and moving with sympathy in every line of his body, Dula took the baby. He met my eyes briefly, questioning, then turned to move through the second set of doors into the high dependency area. There is a flow to admitting a baby, and the room is set up to facilitate that. Immediately through the white doors, recently painted but already flaking a little around the bottom from repeated feet pushing it open, given that often hands are full of babies or supplies, was the weighing area, a set of scales ready with a page of sterilised newspaper on which the baby is placed. Sitting next to that, tucked into the corner, the two open resuscitaires, with heating lamps above, and an oxygen concentrator chugging along below, a tube taking the oxygen to the babies admitted snaking up into each one, secured to the sides with a piece of surgical tape, constantly peeling and being replaced. The sickest babies go here, where they are easily seen and easily accessed. Stretching the length of the room is a series of older incubators, the sides permanently down, despite my repeated attempts to convince the nurses to close them. Dula stopped short just inside the doors, unexpectedly, and I bumped into him while behind, Atsede bumped into me. It would have caused great amusement at any other time, the three of us piling into each other, but the shocked look in Dula's eyes as he turned to look at us quickly put a stop to any inclination to giggle.

As he unbundled the layers of blankets keeping the little baby warm, he had seen the innermost layer, a piece of plastic sheeting, usually wrapped around a stack of *injera* to keep the insects away. While a baby swaddled is a very common sight, even in the warmth of an Ethiopian summer, we were all surprised to see the plastic. But as Dula tried to move it, the reason quickly became apparent. A sharp intake of breath came from over my shoulder, followed a heartbeat later by one of my own, as Atsede and I both saw, for the first time, a baby with the unmistakable diagnosis of epidermolysis bullosa. Shocked, I looked at Dula, whose face mirrored my own. Moving up beside us, Atsede. For one, endless moment, the three of us stood, shoulders touching, in a circle, looking down at the baby, lost for words and hearts breaking. Atsede's eyes filled with tears, and as she gently placed a hand near the baby's head, I heard her murmur a prayer. Dula's voice, deeper and slower, joined in. A breeze came through the cracks in the window, and the baby shifted, unused to the feeling of the open air. As we watched, a piece of the skin on his leg came away, stuck to the plastic. He mewled, the weakest of cries, a result of hours of pain since he was born. Babies with epidermolysis bullosa, the butterfly babies, are missing a key protein responsible for helping the skin to form. Without it, at the lightest touch or the slightest pressure, the skin blisters, cracks, and peels. The severity of the disease varies, but even from just a few minutes of looking, without any diagnostic testing, without so much as touching him, it was clear this baby had experienced one of the nastiest manifestations. At this stage, it was not only his skin that was cause for concern, but also the tissues lining and surrounding his organs, which would be just as susceptible to tearing and fracturing.

In even those few minutes, knowing the agony he must feel was devastating. Seeing suffering, and being unable to do anything to alleviate it, is the single most challenging aspect of clinical care. The hopelessness, the helplessness, is experienced on a fundamental level, deep in our hearts and souls. We are healthcare professionals, a role that becomes a part of our identity, and we are trained and taught how to help, how to heal. But as I looked at Dula and Atsede, I knew that they, like me, were aware there was nothing we could do here for this baby, not really. Our only options would be largely preventative, not even active treatment. Antibiotics could be used to stop an infection, so easily contracted with open sores. IV fluids could avoid dehydration, so likely without the protective barrier of the body's largest organ. Tiny amounts of morphine could be dripped into him, so he wouldn't feel the pain of his skin falling apart. But for all of these we needed a means of administration. I could feel my whole body flinching at just the thought of trying to site a cannula, and then securing it with surgical tape. I could see that Atsede felt the same; she was paler than I had ever known her, and Dula was still standing in exactly the same place, mute now.

'Atsede, I don't know what to do.' My voice was shaking with the effort of controlling my sympathy, not only for the baby, but for his mother. I couldn't imagine how she must be feeling.

'Okay.' It wasn't an agreement; it was a benediction. These were paths we hadn't walked before, and that was okay. I didn't have to have all the answers, all the time, and recognising that was just as important as having a solution. 'Dula?'

The question in her voice, whether he would site the cannula, was met with the shake of his head.

'So, we need Dr Rita.'

The next few hours, and days, were impossible, and yet the minutes ticked by, and the hours passed. We did what we could, and at least, as Atsede tried to reassure us all, time and again, he wasn't in pain. That much we made sure of. When Birabiro took his final breaths, the women of the Neonatal Unit rallied around his young mother, with Zewdu organising endless plates of food and a rota for washing her clothes before she went home later that day.

Even after the beds were cleaned, and the unused morphine vials returned to the pharmacy, carefully checked back in by a staff member with compassion in her eyes as she confirmed we no longer needed them, there was a lingering feeling of failure and sadness. More babies were admitted, more discharged home. Zewdu's son was thriving, and gaining weight before our very eyes, the hollows of his cheeks filling out and rolls starting to form on now-chubby legs. So much life and hope and happiness. And yet, when I looked in the mirror at the end of the day, brushing my teeth, or at Atsede as she reached out to welcome a new baby, or at Dula as I passed him in the corridors, arms full of medical notes or laboratory request forms, it was still haunted eyes that looked back. I knew it would pass; it had done previously, and the resilience of a nurse's morale is striking, but what we needed now was a miraculous save, a chance to stare down the spectre of the memory, not of Birabiro's death, but of his suffering, that hovered over the Unit.

And then Tizazu was born. And then Tizazu survived. Slowly,

the heaviness started to dispel, and our hearts were lighter once more. Birabiro wasn't forgotten, and small paper butterflies, with delicate wings of brightly coloured paper, were now strung across the windows of the Neonatal Unit, and were to stay there for the next four years. Their colours faded in the sunshine of the endless summers, but for those of us who knew the significance, their presence was as vivid as ever. More than six months passed before we picked up the scissors again, and cut new shapes to join the butterflies. But these, starfish this time, weren't a memorial as well as a tribute, and the baby they were created for is now a happy young girl of four.

By this time, much had changed. Tizazu had learnt to sit by himself, smiling and giggling, for his mother the most easily, but over sweet mangoes, watermelon, and papaya too, gifts for him from his doting family, and us, his doting nurses. Atsede and I see him every month or so, for his father, I had found out some weeks after he was discharged from the care of the Neonatal Unit, was the driver for the Dom Boscan Catholic sisters who lived further down our dusty road, and whose borehole we collected water from, 25 litres each day, carried on our backs in the bright yellow jerrycans. Watching him grow, and learn, and play, brought a sense of deep satisfaction and pride in our work, and gratitude to whoever, or whatever, it is that watches over the Neonatal Unit. Atsede had also left the hospital to take up a position leading the Maternal Health Services in a government-run health centre someway away. It was a bittersweet move. We knew the experience would be invaluable for when we opened our own Clinic, but she had been so central to my life at the hospital that the thought of her no longer being there left me somewhat bereft. It was gentle, laughing Selam who stepped into the void Atsede left, both as the senior midwife and as my guide and confidante, and filled it with her quiet humour and affection. I would have been lost without her, and will always cherish the months spent under her tutelage on the night shifts. While Atsede and I are woven from the same cloth, Selam brought an entirely different perspective to life as a midwife, adding a depth and breadth to my understanding of the ways of the Gurage women.

Once again, it was after dusk fell on a day of warm sunshine filling the Delivery Room that Selamawit came, a little nervous, perhaps, but smiling all the same. A midwife, she too had worked here, alongside Atsede, for years before her husband's work took them elsewhere. With Atsede and Selamawit once again on the ward, albeit with Selamawit our charge rather than our colleague and Atsede herself only a month or so from her due date, it was as if, just for this night, we had travelled backwards in time.

After wrapping the worn blood pressure cuff around her upper arm, checking her temperature, and lying her down to find the reassuring thump of her baby's heartbeat, I harried a chatting Atsede and Selamawit out of the heavy wooden doors with strict instructions to keep talking and keep walking. Time seemed to fly by with the usual activity of the Delivery Room. After seeing two women through the operating theatres and into the recovering bay, I made my way to the desk piled high with balls of wool waiting to be crocheted into umbilical cord ties, pinards standing to attention in a line, drying on a square of white cloth, and a haphazard stack of notes. I found Selamawit's, settled into the chair, and spun idly and slowly in a half circle, flicking through her antenatal records and the scan report. Stapled to her blue patient card by Gete, the midwife assisting Dr Rita in the scanning room, nothing stood out particularly. There seemed to be some polyhydramnios, and some placental calcification, but she was now 42 weeks and a few days, so this wasn't that surprising, and certainly wasn't alarming. However, given this, and that she still had no signs of her labour starting, the recommendation from Dr Rita had been for an induction. Selamawit had agreed, trusting Dr Rita, as we all did, and the first dose of the medication used to bring on contractions, misoprostol, had been given at 5pm that afternoon. I glanced up at the clock, frowning with confusion for a few seconds at the time before remembering that the batteries had run out earlier that day. Sighing, yawning, I stood to check the extension cord resting on top of the fridge for an inevitable charging phone. It was now three hours later. I heard a voice call out: it was Zekiya, another of the midwives on duty, needing help. Shifting the notes around,

I managed to find the Delivery Room's only pen, temporarily lost among them, and wrote up my examination of Selamawit, along with the recommendation that she keep mobilising, and return for a foetal heartbeat check in an hour. Spinning on the chair once more – it was a novelty to have a such a chair in the Delivery Room, this one having been borrowed earlier in the day, and we were all making the most of it before the nurses on the ward came to take it back – I got up and made my way around the corner, pushing aside the plaid curtains sewn by the hospital seamstresses.

Zekiya was standing beside the examination couch in the admission room, a stethoscope around her neck and a folded piece of paper in her hand. The woman to whom the paper, a referral letter from a health centre, belonged was on all fours on the bed, swaying her hips from side to side, her eyes closed, her breathing deep and regular.

'Primip from Agena, but hasn't had any ANC, so they don't know her blood. They referred here in case she's negative. Can you type her? And then take her through? I've got ampi and dexa to give.'

This was all said in a language developed by the midwives at the hospital without even realising; a mixture of every day Amharic, English medical terminology, and abbreviations in both, thrown together chaotically. I glanced briefly out of the windows to see if Selamawit and Atsede were making their way back along the corridor, but the world beyond the dense mosquito screens was dark now, the small spheres of light cast by the overhead bulbs only illuminating a small area. I smiled reassuringly at Zekiya.

'Of course, give me the paper.'

Unfolding it, I read through what had been written. It was as I had been told. The woman, Feraworke, was young, or at least she seemed it, and this was her first baby. She hadn't seen a midwife or nurse through her pregnancy, but hadn't reported any problems. Her labour had started around lunch time, and she'd stayed at home until the contractions became too painful to ignore, then had made her way to the nearest health centre. It wasn't unusual for women to have no antenatal care, but if the health centres they then went to in labour didn't have a laboratory working through the night, the nurses automatically sent them to the referral hospital. For women whose blood Rhesus (Rh) factor is negative, an injection of anti-D is recommended after delivery. This is an expensive drug, itself a blood product, costing many thousands of birr and stocked in very few health centres. But it played a crucial role in mitigating the defence systems developed by women's bodies to keep rogue cells in check but which also misidentifies a developing baby as a threat.

Throughout pregnancy the blood flows between a woman and her baby through the veins and arteries of the placenta, bringing oxygen and nutrition, and taking away everything not needed, or wanted, by the growing baby. Sometimes, as part of this process, a few foetal blood cells slip through the mesh, and enter the maternal circulation. If these cells are different from the woman's, in that they are Rh-positive whereas hers are Rh-negative, then they are recognised as foreign, and the woman's body responds as such, creating lifelong memories of them in the form of antibodies. Time passes, and the initial pregnancy ends with the birth of a child, but the antibodies are still there, watching to see that no more of those foreign cells are developing anywhere. If the woman goes on to have another baby with the Rh-positive cells, the antibodies remember. Small enough to pass through the placenta, they seek the source of the remembered cells, and, as is their appointed lot in the immune system, attack them. But these cells aren't bacteria or viruses, vectors of disease, instead they are part of a new, growing baby, and the result is an alloimmune-induced haemolytic anaemia. Mildly affected babies can survive, and are born just a little anaemic or just a little jaundiced. The rich breastmilk of their mother is balm for both, as is sunshine and the passage of time. But for a baby whose blood has been attacked again and again by the antibodies, then there is too much bilirubin produced by the destroyed red blood cells for the placenta to filter, and it builds up in the baby's blood. As the levels rise, this eventually moves across the protective barriers and affects the brain in the form of kernicterus, causing seizures, a loss of reflexes, and a high-pitched, piercingly shrill cry. The outlook for these babies isn't good. Worse yet, another possible outcome is hydrops fetalis, with its cascade of complications, often too much for a tiny body to recover from. The outlook for these babies isn't good either.

It is for this reason that women like Feraworke are referred to a hospital where the miraculous anti-D, which puts a halt to all of this by preventing the memories – the antibodies – from being created in the first place, can be administered if needed. Feraworke's eyes were still closed, but she had stilled, and was resting back on her haunches. I wondered if she was listening. As uncomfortable as she looked, the few minutes between contractions often lulled exhausted women into an in-between world, not quite asleep but not fully awake either. I laid a hand on the small of her back, not wanting to startle her, but needing to move her somewhere safer. The admission room's examination couch was narrow, and covered in bright yellow plastic that quickly became slick with sweat or amniotic fluids.

'Feraworke, can you listen to me for a minute?' She groaned. Whether in response to my question, or to the coming contraction that I could feel tensing the muscles under my hand, I wasn't sure. As it gained in strength, she rocked forward once more, this time her head weaving in time to the low, melodic, whooping that many of the Gurage women make through labour. I looked at Zekiya, who had paused as she walked back through to the room where the antenatal and postnatal women each tried to claim a bed, or half a bed, or a piece of cardboard on the floor. She returned my smile with one of her own, her headed cocked to one side and eyebrows raised. We both sensed that perhaps Feraworke didn't have much longer to go. I didn't think I'd have time for typing, for checking the Rh factor of her blood, after all. It could wait, though the antibodies take time to develop, and we had a window of grace after the birth in which to give it.

As the wave passed, I repeated my question. Feraworke lifted both her eyebrows, her eyes still closed, a silent yes.

'Listen, I'm going to look after you, and help you, but I need you to come with me. This isn't a good place to have your baby.' It was true; I could feel the night's cold breeze coming through the doorway raise goosebumps on my arms. 'But just a few steps this way, it's much better for you. We'll go together. Let's go before the next contraction.'

She came with me, eyes still closed, and not many minutes later I had my hands encased in white gloves, an open aluminium tin on a low wooden stool next to me holding the sterile metal clamps and a pair of scissors. Lying on her side, eyes still closed, her new son slipped easily into my hands, as a gush of clear fluid spilled over the edge of the bed. Uncoiling the cord that had wrapped itself over his shoulder and around an arm as he had turned somersaults while still inside his mother, I placed her tiny baby onto her chest. At last Feraworke opened her eyes, and looked at her child, and smiled.

I still had a smile of my own half an hour later when I heard the rustle of a curtain opening and saw Selamawit and Atsede congregating. I had just finished wiping down the bed, mopping the floors, and cleaning the instruments, and was registering Feraworke's son in the big book kept permanently open on the set of shelves that held the emergency resuscitation equipment.

'You haven't moved in hours, Indie! We've walked how far around the hospital, and you haven't moved.' Atsede's voice was full of mock horror as she sank, with melodramatic flourish, into the spinning chair. Unsurprisisngly, it started to swing with the motion, which Atsede had not been expecting, and she slipped, with very little grace, into a sitting position on the floor. Selamawit and I caught each other's eyes, and burst out laughing. Slapping away the hand I extended to try and help her up a few minutes later, Atsede hauled herself up and tried again, this time sitting more gently. Still chuckling, I turned to Selamawit, and caught her smile just starting to become a grimace. Grinning, I looked at Atsede, who nodded back with pride.

'Yes, it's started! She's been having moderate contractions every couple of minutes for the last half an hour'.

'Good. Stay close then, okay?' I leant over Atsede, receiving a poke in the ribs as I did so, payback for laughing at her, and took one of the pinards from the desk. 'Selamawit?'

She nodded at me, straightening up, and made her way to the place that Feraworke had just left, pulling up her long red dress as she did so. Another contraction came and went, and she stood beside the bed as I knelt and pressed the pinard to the swell of her bump, listening for the steady muffled thud of her baby's heart. As before, it was easy to hear, and low down.

'Keep going, Selamawit. Keep walking, keep talking. Have you got a drink?' She nodded, and motioned to the bag that Atsede had pushed under the desk. 'Good, little sips then, okay? Go on then, and please, take that Atsede with you'. She tried to smile as another contraction started.

Another hour passed, and another, and another, before the tone of Selamawit's groans changed, and the tell-tale sweat started to bead across her brow. As she leaned forward with the latest contraction, she suddenly shifted onto one foot, and Atsede and I, standing and sitting next to her, holding half-empty bottles of Mirinda, the bright orange fizzy drink ubiquitous in birth rooms across Ethiopia, chatting quietly, saw why. Her waters had broken. With that, her baby's head came down further, pressing on the cervix, encouraging those last few centimetres to shift, and open the way. Atsede breathed a quiet whistle: there was a lot of fluid. The diagnosis of polyhydramnios had been accurate, then. Just half an hour later Selamawit was pushing, and we took our positions at her side. Although Atsede no longer worked at the hospital, in the depth of night, with no one else around, and with Zekiya more than happy to sit sipping sweet, spicy tea writing her notes, it was into Atsede's hands that Selamawit pushed her baby.

As she came, Atsede guided her out, and passed the baby up to Selamawit's breast, watching with concern as a larger than normal gush of blood came too. Standing next to her, I placed a hand on top of Selamawit's, which had come up to nestle her daughter, and smiled down, watching happily. Except, in the space of an infinite second, everything changed. Unnoticed by either Atsede, concentrating on the bleeding, or Selamawit, who had her eyes closed from elation, or relief, or both, the baby was struggling. Limp, blue, and silent, she hadn't breathed. Turning her fragile body towards me slightly, I saw the reason instantly. It took a heartbeat to react, reaching, lunging, for the clamps and scissors. With a towel across her tiny torso to keep her warm, I spun and crossed the metres to the neonatal area instantly. Still limp, still blue, still silent. I could feel my own heart beating rapidly in my chest, and the first sensations of real fear creeping around the edge of my mind. The last time I'd felt this way was when I first looked at Birabiro and simply did not know what to do. But this time, I willed myself to calm down, and to methodically go through the stages of neonatal resuscitation that I knew so well. Rub the baby down. Shout for help, if needed. Keep them warm. Check briefly for a heartbeat. Shout for help, if needed. Get the face mask, attached to the bag, which was lying ready in the resuscitation box. Make sure that oxygen is circulating, with chest compressions and puffs of air. Shout for help, if needed.

'Zekiya, if you have a moment, can you come?' Atsede looked up at me sharply, as the creak of Zekiya standing from her chair reached us. 'Now, please.'

I had tried to keep my voice from sounding too afraid. I didn't want to alarm Selamawit, but both Zekiya and Atsede knew from the fear in my eyes that this was a true emergency.

'Oh, God.' The quiet prayer came from Zekiya, now standing next to me, looking down at the still limp, still silent baby, to whom I was giving chest compressions. I tried not to hear her, not to think too much about what it meant, and instead to just move through the motions of resuscitation, an instinctive set of actions, a muscle memory.

'Get the smaller mask for the bag, Zekiya, and help me.' My voice was steadier now. We had performed countless resuscitations before, this was just the same. Except it wasn't. Because this was Selamawit's baby. And because Selamawit's baby was born with a rare genetic condition, undiagnosed antenatally, called Bosma Arhinia Micropthalia, named for the doctor who described it, Bosma, and for its most striking features, arhinia, without a nose, and micropthalia, small eyes. And if I heard Zekiya's plea to God, or thought too much, I would lose the composure I was barely holding together. How could this baby survive? But how could we stop the resuscitation, and allow her to die? Stretching between her eyes was skin and muscle, but no nostrils, no nose, no nasal structures at all. It was a condition, we were later to discover, documented less than 50 times in medical history. Neither Zekiya nor I, nor Atsede, when she stepped up beside us 10 minutes later, after Selamawit's bleeding had settled, to take over the chest compressions, had even heard of the condition, let alone had any idea how to correctly manage a baby with it. But we pushed all of that aside as we continued with the resuscitation.

Yet the unspoken questions were in our eyes in the moments we dared to look at each other. What was going to happen? Were there other, underlying, unknown problems that were also missed? Was this the reason for the later start to her foetal movements early in the pregnancy? And the polyhydramnios at the end? Most of all though, what do we do now? But that, too, was pushed aside as we continued with the resuscitation.

While Atsede and I have both had training in a modified paediatric advanced life support course, given by visiting paediatricians a few months ago, and while the three of us were all certified in the Helping Babies Breathe programme, this was way outside our abilities and knowledge. The problem was, there was no one else. Dr Rita, unusually, was hours away at a meeting in the capital. The only other doctor with any neonatal experience was not on duty, and not on site. We needed a full team of neonatologists, an intensive care unit, paediatric surgeons. All we had was a bag-valve mask, an oxygen concentrator with nasal prongs and a maximum of 5l/min, and a bag of dextrose 40%, sugar water. This hospital is not set up to handle rare and complex neonatal emergencies. This country is not set up to handle rare and complex neonatal emergencies. But she was Selamawit's baby. So we kept going. And we kept going. And when, in the dark night, lit by the ancient stars, her chest rose in a single gasp, relief flooded through us. This was the first step back along the pathway of collapse, away from death and towards life, the first moment of hope, fortifying tired hands and tired hearts. While I couldn't yet let myself believe this story wouldn't end in tragedy, it was an indication that our efforts weren't in vain.

More minutes, more resuscitation, more forcing questions

away. And then, all at once, she cried. As the oxygen flooded her body with each angry sound, her legs curled up, her arms came close to her chest, and the still, silent baby moved with the force of life. The full meaning of that hit us a few moments later. She was alive. Zekiya collapsed back into the chair kept beside the neonatal area, her forehead in her hands, praying quietly under her breath, while Atsede and I remained standing, side-by-side, mute and stunned. Atsede clenched and released her fingers, aching from the compressions and squeezing the bag, and when she raised her eyes to mine, I saw the questions there. Stalling for time, stalling for ideas, I looked around me, trying to find something, anything, to do now. The clink of glass caught my attention, and I glanced down to see where my hands had nudged the tiny vials of vitamin K kept carefully taped to the side of the table. With something tangible to hold on to, but moving as if in a dream, as if the air was thick, I reached for a needle and syringe, drew up the correct dose, and then stood, waiting, wanting someone to tell me whether I should give it or not, whether it was safe, whether we had done the right thing. I couldn't meet Atsede's eye as I raised the syringe to her in an unspoken question. It was just as well, for she couldn't meet mine as she lifted her hands, palm up, and shrugged.

Under the warm glow of the heat lamp, and the rhythm of the rain falling on the tin roof, the baby had just about settled. But as she stopped crying, she stopped breathing. Such a new baby, with nothing but instinct to guide her, relied on being able to breathe through her nose. She had not yet developed the ability to compromise, and so lacked the capacity to utilise the alternative lifeline of breathing through her mouth during moments of calm. In just the few seconds she lay there, suffocating in her own body, her colour started to drain from her fingers, her arms. Without thinking Atsede and I acted at the same time, Atsede reaching for her hand, and me for her foot. We squeezed, gentle at first, then with a little more pressure a heartbeat later, until the baby opened her mouth and cried. The rest of the night stretched out in front of us suddenly as our eyes met. To keep her breathing, we would have to keep her crying, but in doing that she would exhaust herself.

Zekiya, unnoticed by Atsede and I, had found Selamawit's husband, Kibru, sitting in anticipation on the benches outside, where all the men wait for their children to be born, and had brought him through to the Delivery Room. As a nurse himself, he understood better than most the challenges that lay ahead, and we wanted him there as we told Selamawit about her daughter. For the first time, and with some discomfiture at my own feelings, I was grateful that my Guraginya, while passable, was not fluent, because it meant that Atsede would be the one to talk to Selamawit. It would be a difficult, fractured conversation, even given their years of friendship, and I wanted to do something to help. Every time there was a complicated neonatal case, my thoughts returned to Birabiro and his butterflies, and with that, I knew what I could do. Resting my hand briefly on Selamawit's arm, not wanting to interrupt the difficult task that had fallen to Atsede but wanting her to know my heart ached for her, I sidled out of the room and made my way through the rain to the Sister's house.

A few minutes later I returned, my arms wrapped protectively across my chest, keeping the piece of paper I held folded against me dry. Selamawit had turned onto her side, so she could see her baby, still lying under the heat lamp of the neonatal area, now with an oxygen tube taped into place loosely over her open lips. Atsede was at her side, eyes red from the tears that had fallen, but with a determined air. I joined them, unfolding the single sheet of paper. 'Let me show you something. This is a starfish. They too have bright eyes and a smile, but no nose.' Selamawit reached out to touch the buttercup yellow and turquoise blue of the photograph I had printed from the Sister's computer, relieved that they had internet, ink, and power, the only place to do so for hours at this time of night. 'They too are beautiful, Selamawit, and full of life.'

Selamawit kept her fingers on the starfish, and gave the briefest of nods. It was difficult to fathom the turmoil she must be feeling. I looked to Atsede, as I always do, for guidance as to what to do now.

'I think we should add them to the windows. This baby, this Liyu, has a battle to fight, just like Birabiro did.' Atsede had seen my plea and spoke, a sad smile playing over her features as she gave

Selamawit's daughter her name, Liyu, meaning different, special. 'Just like you do, Selamawit.'

While at the Sister's house, I had knocked on the door of another of the nuns, the much-adored and much-respected retired anaesthetist, an eighty-year-old Filipino by the name of Dr Toni who had been at the hospital for over forty years. Hesitant as I was to wake her up, she had been a source of inexpressible comfort and merriment during my time at the hospital, with a no-nonsense, straight-talking attitude that cut through all the uncertainties, and I wanted her help. Although more commonly seen with a screwdriver than a stethoscope, having embraced her new-found interest in the maintenance of the hospital after retiring from clinical practice, with more than four decades of leading the services, she was an invaluable source of knowledge. The last time she had been called to the wards, I tried not to remember, was for a similarly desperate situation, when a woman's blood loss was so significant that her peripheral veins had shut down, her blood retreating within her, keeping what precious little there was perfusing her organs. In that case, Dr Toni had performed what's known as a 'cut down', seeking a vein deep within the woman's leg, cutting through tissue and muscle to find it, exposing the anatomy in a way not often seen outside of an autopsy. A frantic last attempt to keep her circulating volume at a level that would allow her heart to beat. I wondered if she would know of something similar to keep lungs breathing. Moments after I'd finished quietly explaining this to Atsede and Selamawit, the door was pushed open, and in she came.

'Good evening, girls. Indie has told me what's happened. Let me see what we can do to help.' Dr Toni, with a tenderness only seen when she had a baby in her hands, turned Liyu this way and that, fingers gently probing to better feel what bony structures there were, or were not. In the end, despite the decades of experience she could draw upon, Dr Toni had no more answers than we did. She did, however, confirm what Atsede and I had known. We needed to get Selamawit and the baby to Addis Ababa, where – maybe – the answers lay.

'In the meantime, coffee.' I looked at her more closely then, under the harsh lights of the operating theatres that we'd taken Liyu into. Her wrinkled face, so dear to me, was shadowed with tiredness.

'Dr Toni, I'm so sorry for waking you. Of course, we'll make coffee.' She cackled like a *jereba*, the jackals that circle the town, at that. Surprised, I smiled in question.

'Not for me! I'm not so old that I need coffee to stay awake in the night.' She raised an eyebrow in challenge as I opened my mouth to tease her about her age, as I had so often done before. 'For the baby. Coffee stimulates the respiratory systems, at least in preterm babies. We could try it. It will unsettle her, but it might keep her breathing. Prepare just a small *sini*, like normal, and add half a ml as she breastfeeds, every time she comes off to breathe, give a drop.'

After walking Dr Toni back through the night to the convent, holding my arm out for her to take, knowing she finds the uneven ground difficult in the dark, I relayed the suggestion to Atsede. Shrugging, she agreed, willing to try anything.

The months, and then the years, passed. And Liyu survived. And so did Selamawit. Not a single day has been easy, she said to us as we celebrated Liyu's third birthday with lukewarm Fanta and thick, freshly baked bread, but not every day is hard. There had been an incredible chance, a year or so ago, to travel to the capital to meet with an internationally renowned specialist in cranio-facial abnormalities, arranged through the serendipitous, gracious work of Dr Natalie Shaw from the Clinical Research Branch of NIHS. We had gone, nervous but hopeful, spending an anxious two nights at the convent of the Franciscan Missionaries of Our Lady while we waited for the meeting, for the results of scans, for a plan. There wasn't much that anyone could do with Liyu so young, and with so many unknowns, but the gentle, assured natures of Dr Gravem and Dr Mekonnen, and the knowledge that we had managed to successfully arrange this extraordinary meeting, was a balm for Selamawit. Even without any certain answers, for the simple fact that there were none, Selamawit had said that just knowing there was a team of experts who were aware of Liyu, and that they had guaranteed to us that they would do what they could to help, made her feel less alone.

Atsede

The wooden door swung open suddenly, catching me by surprise, and I felt myself jump before turning to see who it was appearing so dramatically. Indie. I smiled in greeting, catching the tell-tale glint of determination in the set of her mouth, and wondered what she had been up to.

'Konjo, peace. Where have you been! It's late, rounds have finished, there's work to do.' It was true, I had looked for Indie all over the hospital before gathering up the medical notes of the women to be seen, throwing open the windows to bring in the morning sunshine, and introducing myself to the families and friends gathered around each bed, sipping *kawa* and eating *kolo*, roasted barley.

'Atse, good morning. What are you doing? Are you busy?'

'Atsede, peace.' Selam had followed her through the doors, and was now grinning exasperatedly at Indie, who hadn't waited for my answer, but instead manoeuvred herself behind me and was checking through the treatment plans devised by Dr Rita for the high-risk women expected to birth in the coming hours. I just opened my mouth in response, when Indie spoke up again.

'Ah, not so busy then, Atse. *Ishi,* okay, let's go.' And with that, Indie slipped her arm into mine, and what felt like only moments after she and Selam had first appeared, I was guided back out of the wooden door and into the bright sunshine. Laughing, I turned to Indie.

'What is going on, Indie? Where's the emergency?' Indie avoided answering, harrying us ahead of her instead. Turning to me, Selam raised her eyebrows and shrugged at my question, with just as little idea as I had as to why we were being steered along the shady veranda. Monkeys jumped from the trees either side of us, curious eyes watching our progress, the sound of their feet clattering over the corrugated iron, as we made our way towards the benches outside the Neonatal Unit.

'Why do I get the feeling we might be about to find out where she's been all morning, Selam?' I muttered, glancing back over my shoulder just in time to see Indie roll her eyes. A minute later, as I expected, we stopped abruptly in front of the peeling, cracked red paint of the Neonatal Unit.

Turning to face us, motioning that we sit, I watched as Indie took a breath.

'Atse, Selam, I need you to help me.' Indie's voice was steady, but her hands were clenched at her side, a sign I knew only too well. It meant I wouldn't like whatever I was about to be asked to do. Indie, having sat us down just moments beforehand, now beckoned for us to stand, and pointed through the window. 'Tizazu's haemoglobin has dropped again, and his markers are up. I'm worrying. His head circumference has stopped increasing, but there's a lot of blood in that haematoma that now isn't in his circulating volume.'

'He's O neg, isn't he.' It was said more as a statement than a question. Selam, who had been there for his birth, and had been with Indie when the initial diagnosis was made, knew Tizazu's case well. I sighed. Of course, he was O negative. The same as Indie. Which meant...

'I can give.' Indie said, finishing my thought out loud. She glanced sheepishly at me, knowing already that I would have reservations. She has asked me a thousand times why I won't give blood, never, apparently, receiving a satisfactory answer. The truth is at the same time so simple, and so complex, as is often the way. I am afraid. Not of the momentary sting of a needle, but of the simple fact that I can never know what is coming. I have worked too long in the hospital, seeing the cases coming through the Emergency Room and the Delivery Room, to believe without some doubt that I will survive tomorrow, or the day following that, or the day following that, without accident or injury. I am afraid that perhaps something will happen, and I will need every drop of blood in my veins to stay alive. Even if not me, then my family, my sisters, my brothers. If I give blood today, what's to say I won't regret it tomorrow? But I can't ever seem to find the words for my fears, instead relying on silence to keep them at bay, as if speaking it out loud would be a malediction. Lost in thought, I only half listened to Indie's explanations. In my mind, I could already play out the scenes that would come. I would argue my corner, she would argue hers, and neither of us would change our minds. Selam, the voice of reason, as she has been before, would mediate. Sure enough, almost exactly as I had imagined, I found myself asking Indie to reconsider, then listening to Selam find the middle ground, then watching Indie promise not to give blood for three months as long as we helped Tizazu now. I smiled, as much at my own prescience as at Indie's barely concealed delight that she had convinced us.

With the notes already gathered, and the results from the most recent blood tests taken just a few hours earlier (an answer to Indie's absence this morning, as I had suspected) in hand, Indie blew us a kiss and turned to go, determined to find Dr Rita and get her plan into action before either Selam or I could find a reason to back down. A few steps later, she turned back abruptly, and handed over a sheaf of papers.

'Homework, children. Read these, please.' It was said as a mock command, but the creases at the corners of her eyes showed she was full of gratitude. Her tone softened, and I saw how much she wanted this to work. 'Information on direct blood transfusions. We'll need to work it all out on paper before we do it for real.'

I raised my hands in exasperation, turning to Selam in disbelief. 'First she press-gangs us into helping her, and now she's giving us homework! Be careful, Indie, I'm onto you.' Selam's laughter dampened the impact of my dire threat, and was soon joined by the chattering of the monkeys as Indie passed by their trees once more on her way to find Dr Rita.

'It was inevitable, Atse. You know how she is once she's made her mind up. It's been difficult, for all of us, since Birabiro. She needs this.' Selam laid a reassuring hand on my forearm as I winced at hearing his name. It seemed incredible that almost a month had already passed. Time had thrown itself ahead since he died. More and more often now, the days seem to go by without me thinking of him, except when I go to the Neonatal Unit, of course, where the paper butterflies still dance. But now Selam had said his name, it all came flooding back.

I remember the evening he was admitted with almost painful detail. Bearing witness to sadness is as much a part of midwifery as bearing witness to happiness. It isn't so much that I've become impervious to either, but more than I've found a way to keep going despite them. In the same way that I would wear dark colours or talk about a donkey while with a *Budah* sorceress, to protect my mind from their unconscious malicious powers during a visit, I've learnt there are ways to shield my heart from the impact of the river of emotions that comes with all I witness during a birth. But there are times sadness breaks through. After all, the smoke of *chaniya*, of rue, can't keep all the *bimbi*, the mosquitoes, away. And actually, I don't mind still feeling sadness when thinking of Birabiro. His memory deserves that.

His mother will still be *chyne*, in the months after a birth where the woman stays mostly in her room, resting her body, familiarising herself with her new role in life, her new baby. Birabiro's mother will sleep alone, though, without the warmth of her son next to her. I felt the sadness wash over me again. I had seen sisters, cousins, friends experience this. The language we use is the same for women who have a baby in their arms as for those whose babies live only in their hearts. The *chyne* is the same too. The women rest their minds – their hearts – as much as their bodies, trying to come to terms with what has happened to them, what has happened to so many of the women who came before them, and the ones before them. Those coming to visit take a seat on the wooden *burchama* stools set out alongside the mattress, and listen to the story of what happened, lament with the mother, trying to offer a little comfort. For Birabiro's mother – I can't believe I have forgotten her name already – the comfort would be hard to come by. Despite the warmth of the sunshine, the sounds of laughter from convalescing patients enjoying a little respite on the grass, and the knowledge that we were about to help Tizazu, I felt a shiver pass through me. I've helped to bring babies into this world different in all kinds of ways, it is simply a part of caring for women with almost no chance to see a midwife in their pregnancy, but seeing Birabiro was no easier for that. Epidermolysis bullosa, Indie said it was called, as if giving it a name might help us understand what to do. But how could anyone understand what to do with a baby whose own skin is falling apart? How do you offer comfort to the baby, to the mother, when the only ways you know how to do that – touch, warmth, closeness – cause nothing but suffering? In the end, we could do only what nurses and midwives everywhere do: we cared. The morphine we dripped into his tiny vein via a cannula that only Dr Rita had the strength of spirit to site, and site again when the plaster holding it in place fell away with the skin of his scalp, kept him free of pain. But from the moment we first gave it, Birabiro was in a world inbetween, never awake, nor really asleep. He was in limbo. From the moment he was born, really. And when he died, his mother thanked Allah for, at last, releasing him from his suffering. She mourned his loss, but not his death. Indie has been telling me the tales from her country, the 'great love stories' she calls them, written by people long ago with names like Shakespeare and Woolf, but they always seem to be about a man and a woman. If I were going to write a great love story, well, that wouldn't be who I would write about. In my mind, the tales of true love, surely, are the ones about mothers and their children. In no other circumstance will you see such selfless, self-sacrificing, unconditional love. Many years ago, before the hospital came, when there was no recourse for newborns too sick or too small to survive, it was the women called upon to leave these babies by the river, where the *gwencha,* the hyenas, congregated at dawn and dusk. Only in motherhood do you see such emotion. In Guraginya, my language, we talk of pregnant women as *hwetawrra,* as having two souls. Hers, of course, and her child's. For that unique handful of months of a pregnancy, she carries two souls within her, two perfect, untarnished souls, before releasing one, in a whirlwind of pain and power, into the world. Now, if that isn't the start of a great love story, I don't know what is. What other experience could possibly be as intense, as challenging, as affirming, as that?

We, as Birabiro's clinicians, not his family, continued to reel from the feelings of hopelessness, of knowing that, no matter how much we wanted it, we couldn't prevent his own body's betrayal. It made sense to me that Selam was connecting Tizazu's case to Birabiro, regardless of how dissimilar they might seem at first. As if she knew she'd slipped into my thoughts, Selam spoke up again.

'Anyway, you know who Tizazu's father is, don't you?'

My interest piqued, I turned to her. 'No?'

'Nardos. The driver from the Catholic order.' It clicked in my mind. I recognised his wife, and even, now I knew, thought there was something of Nardos's features in the soft curves of Tizazu's face.

Working for any of the Catholic orders was a good position to have, with a reliable salary and, often, small items no longer needed at the houses gifted to the staff. Nardos was a good man, a good husband, and he would be a good father to Tizazu. I had heard him speak of his work with the priest; he enjoyed the opportunity to travel the area, visiting the churches, meeting with the parishioners. There have been Catholic nuns and monks here for as long as anyone can remember, and many families in my village have been Christian for generations. Looking at the sandstone walls of the hospital around me, and through the trees and bushes to Lorde Mariam, the church built adjacent, I sat back against the cool bench, closing my eyes, and let my mind wander.

Faith is woven through my life, from the childhood years spent running barefoot through the church, collecting flowers for the altars or chasing errant goats away, to the thoughtful hours meeting with Abba, the priest, before my wedding. Even in the darkest of moments, the most difficult of days, the teachings that suffering can be met with courage, hate with love, and anger with acceptance, I find of inexpressible comfort. The same comfort that those with faith have felt all over the world, and all through time. Here, in Ethiopia, Christianity is ancient, as old as the Testaments themselves. They even say the Ark of the Covenant is here, brought to its final resting place from a sacked Jerusalem by Menelik, the son of the Queen of Sheba and King Solomon, and has remained hidden in the cool depths of a rock-hewn church in Aksum ever since, guarded by warrior priests who train their entire life for the task. Then again, just as many people say this isn't true, and that the Ark was lost or destroyed or never existed in the first place. Whatever the truth is, perhaps it doesn't matter: perhaps the comfort from believing in it is enough.

I opened my eyes at the harsh caw of a marabou, nesting in the bell tower of the church. My eyes were drawn to the stained-glass windows, and the door standing ajar. The church, like the hospital, never closed. Both were built, decades ago, by the Medical Missionary Sisters, a Catholic order of clinically trained nuns, who have intertwined their devotion to God with their dedication to healing His people. I smiled gently to myself, remembering the time not that long ago when I had every intention of joining them. I liked, and still like, the idea of spending my life in service to others. But over time I came to realise I saw God not in hours of quiet contemplation, but in the laughter of my friends, in the love of my nieces and nephews as they look at their mother, in the songs and drumbeats and dancing of the hymns, and, above all, in my work as a midwife, in the miraculous moments of life and death I witness there.

Next to me, Selam stood, stretching and yawning. She'd been up most of the night with her son Tensu no doubt, and gathered up papers Indie had left, before motioning back towards the Delivery Room.

'I'll come in a moment. All the notes are on the desk, and Dr Rita has been through already. The midwives today are Dage and Tamrat, both with the two women with contractions.' I smiled as she left, her long green dress swishing around her ankles as she pulled on her white gown again, checking its pockets for something or other before looking at the papers in her hands. I sat back again, enjoying the warmth of the sunshine before it became too hot. The clank of a trolley, and call of the staff working in the sterilising rooms echoed down the veranda, and I glanced up the length of it, wondering if Indie had finished with Dr Rita, but there was no sign of her yet, so I too stretched and stood, and started back.

'Atse!' It was Selam, rounding the corner and almost colliding with me, 'Oh, you're coming. Listen, I've just flicked through our homework from Indie. I imagine Dr Rita will agree, so we'll be doing venous to venous, *ishi*, which means we're going to need to work out how long we've got before the blood will clot.' I nodded in agreement. 'So, let's practise. If we get some syringes, we can take a little from Indie and then just time it through a 3ml, a 5ml, and a 10ml.'

'Here?'

'No, let's go back to the Neonatal Unit. Do you want to make sure everything is under control here, and meet me there? Hopefully we'll pick up Indie on the way.'

Another nod and Selam left, stopping briefly at the long wooden shelves that held the supplies for the Delivery Room, collecting, no doubt, syringes, tourniquets, and gloves.

'Dage!' I called out, wandering into the staff area, and found Dage trying to balance a big, dented aluminium tin across a camping stove. Filled with water, and the submerged rubber tubing from the obstetric vacuum, it would sterilise the bits of equipment that couldn't handle the high heat of the autoclave standing next to it. 'There's been a vacuum?'

'Peace, Atesde. No, well, almost, but in the night. Failed vacuum, she went for CS.' We both winced on behalf of the woman.

'*Ishi*, well, thank you for sorting the tubes out. I'm going with Selam to the Neonatal Unit for an hour or so. Everything okay here?'

'Oh, yes'. Dage, having finally balanced the tin, turned to face me, peeling off the blue gloves and throwing them into the bucket under the desk, before leaning back against the autoclave. The warmth from it lasted hours after the sterilisation stopped, and was always a favourite spot to rest. 'She said. You're transfusing Nardos's child? It's a good idea, that haematoma looked bad even yesterday.'

'Mm. Indie is with Dr Rita now.'

'*Ishi*. Go. Everything is fine, here.'

One last glance through the windows into the adjacent room, where the women who delivered in the night were sitting, or dozing, with their newborns tucked in close. It all seemed calm. Walking back through the swinging wooden doors, I heard my name being called. It was Indie, looking satisfied, motioning for me to wait for her.

'Atse, are you running away? Too late now. Dr Rita is just finishing up with the cervical cancer screening, and then she's coming too.' She smiled at me. 'Thank you, Atse, for agreeing to help. I know you don't agree.'

'Indie, it isn't that I don't agree. I want to help Tizazu as much as you do. You just have to look after yourself too! Like Selam said, you can't give all your blood away. You'll be no use to me at all if you're all dried up.'

She laughed. 'I've already promised. Not another drop for three months.' Tugging on the sleeve of my white coat, we started towards the Neonatal Unit. 'Except the mosquitoes' share, of course!' It was said ruefully, as Indie slapped her arm suddenly. 'In the daytime, Atsede, that's not acceptable. If my haemoglobin drops, it's because of these mosquitoes. They are the work of the Devil.'

'You may be right there. Enough playing, let's go give that baby some blood.'

Minutes later, everything was set up. Selam had found a clean cloth and a clock, and had set the syringes out. It looked something like an altar, I thought to myself. With Indie sitting down, we started, taking a little blood in each syringe, and timing ourselves as we pushed it out, waiting until the clotting started. It reminded me so much of the days in the past where I had done just this to diagnose DIC, disseminated intravascular coagulopathy. For women who have been bleeding too much for too long, eventually their blood simply runs out of the protein necessary to stop it. When that happens, there's nothing left, no platelets, no clotting factors, and the bleeding continues. It happens in women with infections, with pre-eclampsia, with placental abruption. When these women start bleeding from their cannulation sites, or from any small injuries, or vaginally if their have already delivered their baby, I take a syringe of blood and sit, waiting minutes for it to clot, then push the plunger only to see it drip out easily on the piece of gauze lying waiting, and I know this is the problem. As with the name for Birabiro's condition though, knowing it's DIC doesn't necessarily mean knowing the next step in management.

Needing to know is such a fundamental human trait. We always want to know, to know what happened, to know what to do next, to know what will come, to know how to stop it. That must be why the *wog* is always greeting guests. As the authority on Gurage folklore and tradition, it is the *wog* who offers answers to these questions, always steeped in the archaic knowledge of the Gurage people. I remembered Abe, the young man little more than a boy from the compound next to my family's, who accidentally killed a stray cat when a stone thrown to discourage it from stealing meat from the blackened pot sitting waiting to go on the fire was a little too accurate and a little too hard. This marked the start of his descent into madness, according to the *wog,* which culminated, days later, in his unexpected death, hanging from a tree in the garden. It was because he killed the cat, the *wog* had said; it upset the natural order, the delicate balance of life. Animals are not killed here for anything less than food, which is a necessity for survival. Even hyenas wandering too close to the huts, taking goats and chickens, are not hunted. In any case, it is well known that if you kill one, his family will take revenge. When Abe killed the cat, he didn't tell anyone, so there was no chance for the community to gather and offer placating prayers and apologies, washed down with *kawa* and *kollo*. But the *wog* knew. Just as he knew what Abe's family needed to do afterwards, to put things right, to restore the equilibrium, to prevent the madness from taking them all. A sheep must be slaughtered, the *wog* had said, and the blood collected, then given to the all the wild cats. That is the apology, for the loss of one of them at the hands of one of us. Then, to prevent any lingering evil, each member of the family must take the water and *kemem*, spices, used to prepare the *jebena,* the black clay *kawa* pots, and wash their hands with it, every day for seven days. This will protect them. Indie and I had been at the *luxor*, the mourning, for Abe. His family lived next to mine, our huts, our gardens, our lives, separated only by the wooden posts dug into the ground that served as a fence. Whether or not I believed in what the *wog* had deemed necessary was unimportant. I saw the comfort it brought to the family, in having answers, in knowing.

And now we knew too, how long we had before Indie's blood would coagulate in the syringe. Just in time, with Dr Rita arriving at the door, her instantly recognisable white scrubs already crinkled after she'd spent the morning standing and sitting by the side of the narrow cot that served as the examination couch in the consultation room. She smiled in greeting at all of us, then crossed the small room and sat on the huge concrete block that, inexplicably, took up a quarter of the space in there. It served as a good place to store things, but made moving around difficult. I remembered when this had been the laundry room, long before I worked here, but in the days when my father was a nurse's aide, and I came to bring him lunch, or visit briefly after school. The concrete block was built so the washerwomen had a place to scrub the clothes, and after the laundry block had been moved to its new site, and the Neonatal Unit started here, it hadn't been worth the work to remove it. So it stayed.

With Dr Rita here, we could begin. I felt Indie flinch, and close her eyes momentarily, as the needle of the cannula broke through the soft skin of her inner elbow. It was with relief that I saw the bright red blood flood into the tiny tube. I didn't often miss a vein, but was pleased nonetheless. I motioned for Indie to drop her arm to her side, so gravity could work in our favour to keep the blood flowing. Because of the timing of the clotting, balanced against the time it took to gently push Indie's blood into Tizazu's even tinier tube, we would have to keep the cannula working. They are designed to keep an access point into a vein, so drugs and fluids can be given over days, but aren't always so great at allowing blood to be taken from them. For now, though, with Indie slowly clenching and releasing her fist, there was almost enough in the first syringe.

I turned to Selam, standing relaxed next to me, her hands encased in white sterile gloves clasped in front of her, talking easily with Tizazu's mother, then looked to Dr Rita, sitting behind them, and nodded. 'Syringe one, ready.'

'Okay. Selam, ready?' Dr Rita stayed where she was, but leaned forward slightly, watching closely as I passed the syringe across to Selam, and Selam connected it to Tizazu's cannula, matching

Indie's in the crook of his arm. Slowly, steadily, Selam pushed the plunger, and we watched, holding our breath, as the syringe emptied out. Again, and again, and again we repeated this, not saying much more than 'Ready? ready' in all the minutes we were there, until the final syringe was emptied.

'*Ishi*, finished. Well done, Selam, Atsede. Indie, will you keep me updated on how he is? Repeat bloods tomorrow morning, give his medicine as before. Mama, let him nurse and sleep like normal. Thank you, everyone. Good work.' Dr Rita stood to leave, nodding at us, and extracting a pen clipped to the front of her scrubs to sign Tizazu's medical notes, confirming what she had just told Indie. Having a cannula in place is not comfortable for anyone, but particularly for a newborn who can't understand why it's there. Despite that, though, he had cried very little, and was now back at his mother's breast, exactly where he belonged. Selam and Indie were watching, smiling gently, Indie with a piece of gauze held over the tiny hole in her skin left behind by the cannula.

'Selam, Indie, who wants to stay here? And who is coming to Delivery?' They glanced at each other.

'I'll stay.' It was Indie, as I had expected. Giving Selam a little shove, she settled back onto the chair, checking to see the bleeding had stopped at the cannula site. 'Thank you, both of you.'

With that, Selam and I edged past the plastic cot, and made our way back through the warm sunshine to Delivery, talking happily. It may have been on that walk, or one of the many others to and from the Neonatal Unit that we took over the following weeks as we checked on Tizazu's progress, that Selam and I found out that our friend, Selamawit, was *hwetawrra*, expecting a baby. It is usual for young women here to marry and have children, so while bringing great happiness, it wasn't such a surprise. Nor, really, was it such a surprise when, just a few days after Selamawit had a positive pregnancy test, I too found out that the tiredness and nausea I had simply put down to a relapse of P. vivax (malaria), which happened almost yearly, in fact had another cause altogether. I hadn't even thought to put a circle around 'HCG' when sending off the vial of blood Tagesh had taken from me during a lull in births. But when

Hailu came to hand over the results for all the blood tests from Delivery that day, there it was, scribbled in blue pen with a small exclamation mark, 'positive!'. I had groaned with dismay at that, not realising that one word which would change my life was written not next to the P. vivax box as it looked at first glance, but a little way further down the piece of paper. The exclamation mark struck me as odd though. Malaria is a common disease to have. Nearly everyone I know has spent days in bed, sweating and shivering with a pounding head and aching joints. It was that exclamation mark that had me looking a little closer, tracing my finger from the 'positive!' to the left, and seeing it there, in printed black letters, 'HCG'. Even then it took a moment to realise. But when I did, I could feel my mouth drop open and my heart start to pound. Positive. I was pregnant. I touched my stomach, marvelling already at the tiny little baby inside. Dawit and I had married six months ago, so it wasn't unexpected. But, my God, pregnant. I would be a mother. I laughed out loud, startling the family members sitting with a woman who had birthed in the night on the other side of the curtain. Looking more closely, I recognised the writing as that of my cousin, a laboratory technician who had started at the hospital not long after I had, and smiled, pleased because I knew that meant the news wouldn't spread quickly around the hospital. She would keep it quiet.

'Tagesh!' I called out. Her head appeared around the corner, a blood pressure cuff and stethoscope in her hand. 'Tag, when you sent my bloods, you requested HCG as well?'

She grinned sheepishly. 'Really, Atsede. How are you our *halafi*, our manager? You have nausea, tiredness, and achiness, and are a healthy young woman just married? "Malaria", you said. Honestly, what kind of a midwife...'

'*Ishi*, you. Don't even get me started on how many ethical lines you've just crossed. Consider this a warning not to do that to anyone else.' Though I meant it, and indeed later Tagesh did come to apologise for her presumption and admitted she would never have done it with anyone else, I couldn't help smiling at the results. I told Dawit a few days later, one evening as we were lying in bed, watching the mosquitoes land on the outside of the *angoba,* the net, trying to find a way in. Pleased with the news, he congratulated me, and solicitously asked after my health, before the conversation turned elsewhere. I told Indie the next day, one afternoon as we navigated the holes and resting livestock strewn across the dirt track on the way to the market. Her shriek of delight before picking me up, clear off the ground, and whirling me around were not entirely what I expected. I read an article recently about generational trauma, how our bodies remember the challenges and distress of our forebearers on a cellular level. Their ordeals actually change their DNA, which is then passed on to their children, and their children's children, a chemical epigenetic scratch that can be traced back through the decades. When I think of Indie's reaction compared to that of my Gurage friends, I can believe it. So many of our babies die, in pregnancy, in childbirth, in the first years of life, and during those 1,000 days when a child's hold on life is tenuous, that I think now my contemporaries and I have changed from the cumulative effects of heartbreak. I was happy, deeply happy, to be pregnant, but also wary of believing that meant, without doubt, I would have a child at the end of it. And it wasn't a choice to feel that way, not something that I could control; instead it just was. I was afraid of tempting fate, afraid to get caught up in the joy in case it ended in sadness. As physiology influences behaviour, behaviour influences culture. Selamawit and I spoke about it, I remember, as our stomachs swelled with our unborn children. When we sat, drinking *kawa,* eating lunch, comparing how difficult we were finding it washing clothes in the river, carrying jerrycans of water, chopping wood, we also wondered if our pregnancies would give us a child. Like almost everyone I've known, we didn't prepare clothes, choose a name, or discuss the babies themselves.

Now, it is so ingrained in our culture to wait until the birth to believe you've made it through, that Indie's transparent, undoubting exuberance was jarring. Even with her experiences as a midwife, seeing the best and worst of birth every day, she never doubted that I and my baby would be okay. I didn't ask Dawit for a name for our son until he was a few days old, but I did allow

Indie to bring a blanket and baby clothes from England when she went to visit during the middle of my pregnancy. And then, three years later, when once again the tiredness, aching, and nausea took over my mornings, and my son was to have a younger sibling, I found myself, somehow, caught up in Indie's determination to choose the perfect name, whether I had a boy or a girl. Indie and I lived together now, spending all our time never more than a stone's throw apart, so I couldn't help but be infected by her enthusiasm. It took her weeks, and many conversations with all manner of people about the meanings behind all her possibilities, but she did it, and Natnael was named weeks before he was born, a fact that took my own mother by great surprise. I think about that now and wonder if, in the same way that our DNA can be scratched in the past, it can be healed in the present.

Then again, the scratch is deep here. Even now, many women, and many, many babies don't survive. Or they do, but are left with almost insurmountable challenges. I don't have to look any further than Selamawit, one of my closest friends, to be reminded of that. Around the same time that I was walking with Selam to and from the Neonatal Unit, watching delightedly as Tizazu's haematoma shrank, as his colour came back, as the lab reports tucked away in his medical notes showed a rising haemoglobin, I also sat at the bedside of Selamawit's older sister as she pushed her silent baby into the world. It is a privilege to care for these women, the women whose babies will never cry, the ones the mothers have to say goodbye to without ever having the chance to say hello, but also a heavy responsibility. Even if neither they, nor you, realise it at the time, every word you say, the comfort you try to offer, stays with them. I've had so much practice, so many years, of offering comfort, that I know what to say now. I tell them what I learnt at school. That energy cannot be created or lost, it is simply moved around between everything that has ever, and will ever, exist in this world. That their child shared in that, they had some of that energy within them, it moved their blood around their body, and kept them warm and growing. That energy still exists: maybe not all together now, but it still exists somewhere. I tell them that their baby played a part in the movement of energy through time and place. I don't expect it to make the women feel better, necessarily, but I do hope that they remember those words, one day, and remember that their baby mattered, not only to them, but to the existence of everything. Selamawit's sister, Meskerem, had said very little, both during the birth and afterwards. But then again, some people survive hardship and talk about it. Some people survive and don't. And all people deal with unimaginable pain in their own way. The last thing I said to Meskerem, before she left after the burial of her son, was to remember how big the sky is, and to know, that just because there are storms here now, it doesn't mean there isn't sunshine on the horizon. The winds will blow and take the clouds, and the warmth will come back. Maybe not tomorrow, maybe not this month, but it will.

Sitting at the bedside of Selamawit herself, several months later, less than a handful of weeks from my due date, I was reminded, once more, of the fragility of certainty. The months of her pregnancy had given us no reason to believe that the hours of her labour would be anything other than straightforward, nor the growth and movements of her stomach an indication there would be anything other than a healthy baby at the end. The first, at least, was true. By the time Selamawit had passed 41 weeks, there was still no sign that her body was preparing for labour. With all that is known about the human body, the mysteries of childbirth remain elusive still. As the days kept passing by, Selamawit took the advice of the women, lighting a fire and balancing a blackened pot full of water and ground grains on three rocks. *Telba* has been made here for generations as a way to gently coax in labour, or to persuade hesitant tightenings into a regular pattern of contractions. Sweetened with freshly harvested honey, and sipped throughout the day, the *telba* Selamawit made was kept warm on the coals for days, until, nearing 43 weeks, I met her at the roadside, ready to go together to the hospital. She had come to my house just the afternoon before, arriving as Indie and I sat cross-legged on the floor, arguing over who had cheated in the most recent game of cards. The windows and doors were thrown open in an attempt to bring in some breeze, and there was a growing pile of *gishte,* custard apple, skins and seeds next to us. It was a Sunday, and Indie had spent the weekend at my house. It was almost four months since I had finished my last shift at the hospital. Instead, I worked at Amorameda, a government-run health centre. It was different, and leaving the hospital woven into so much of my life took time to adapt to, but as the weeks of my pregnancy passed, I appreciated the slower pace of life there.

It had become a habit for Indie to spend the weekends with me, and we both enjoyed the time together as I showed her life away from the hospital where, until now, she had spent all of her time. Saturdays these days found us at weddings, funerals, christenings, feast days, and celebrations, Sundays at church, at my family compound, ringed with *sahrbet* huts in Sisa, the village, at my home in the town, roasting *kawa,* learning to cook *habersha* dishes, and playing endless games of cards. With the constant exposure to the dialect of Guraginya spoken by my family and friends, rather than the Ethiopian's lingua franca, Amarinya, spoken in the hospital, her understanding improved fast, helped in no small part by my mother, who would only speak to her in our language, expecting her to respond in kind and scolding her if she didn't.

If I was covering the weekend at Amorameda, Indie joined me there instead, another pair of gloved hands to help out in the Emergency Room or MCH Services. In the evenings, the guards would build a bonfire, and she sat with us as we teased, told stories, and ate *shunkura,* sugar cane. After midnight, when the patients stopped coming, we pulled down the woven mats from where they were stored on top of the medication cupboards and slept together under thick blankets, mosquito nets strung up between a nail in the wall and the handle of the window. As well as the simple pleasures of friendship and camaraderie, my time at Amorameda was also invaluable experience in the management of a health facility. Not very many months later, this would be my new role, with Atsede's Clinic opening its doors for the first time.

Before that time came, though, there were weekends to fill, and games of cards to play, and babies to be born. First, Selamawit's, then my own, then my sister's. That Sunday, we had teased Selamawit about how she had adopted the swaying, side-to-side walk of a pregnant woman, and laughed at the look of evident relief that came when she could sit, leaning against the high back of the wooden chair, the swell of her abdomen seemingly huge. Indie and I shifted from our places on the floor, finding stools to sit on and a crate that could serve as a table. Another hand was dealt, and as we flipped over cards, Selamawit told us she had been to the hospital yesterday, and met with Dr Rita for an ultrasound. Glancing at the clock that my younger brother had given to me, a wedding gift, I made to get up, my own swollen abdomen getting in the way a little. Indie sat, head cocked to one side, watching my struggle with poorly concealed amusement.

'*Dredig, dredig*', I heard her say, slapping the back of one hand against the palm of the other, a Gurage gesture expressing her despair at what she was witnessing. 'This is too sad to watch Atse, you can't even stand up anymore. And yet you still won't ask for help. Selamawit, what should we do? Leave her?' Selamawit laughed before running a hand over her own bump. I grinned at them both before motioning for a hand.

'*Ishi*, Indie. Stop talking and help me. We have *bazhara*, guests, and we haven't even served *kawa* yet. Have I taught you nothing about Gurage hospitality? This is unacceptable.'

Sighing, I watched as Indie put her arm around Selamawit. 'Selamawit isn't really a guest, though, is she? She's our family. Still, you're right. It's time for *kawa*.' Indie stood, stretching her hands in front of her dramatically. 'It's time. And I will do it! I will make amazing *kawa*.'

Trying not to laugh, I turned to Selamawit. 'Are you ready for this? I have been teaching her every weekend, but this is the first time Indie will make it alone.'

Selamawit threw a glare in my direction before turning to Indie, smiling kindly. 'You can do it Indie. Wash the beans well, don't roast them too much, and make sure the *jebena* is hot before you add them.'

Smiling gratefully at the advice, Indie turned to me, pulling a face, before making her way through the open doorway to the mud-caked walls of the wooden kitchen behind the house.

While the sounds of Indie washing, roasting, and pounding the *kawa* filtered through, Selamawit and I discussed what Dr Rita had said. Indie reappeared briefly, bringing cool glasses of water poured from the jerrycan she'd brought from the Sister's house that morning, a cause of great entertainment for the women gathered at the pumps, before disappearing back outside.

It was nothing we hadn't expected, really. Now approaching 43 weeks, Selamawit's placenta had started to calcify, and there was a question about polyhydramnios. But otherwise, *hulum selam,* all was at peace, there were no problems. She was to go again, the next day, to decide with Dr Rita what to do next. She was a little apprehensive – I knew her well enough to hear it in her voice – but also ready for her pregnancy to be over. The last week, she said, had been difficult. Even just moving around, she was tired. Selamawit had been my friend for many years, and looking at her closely, I could see the smudges of darkness under her eyes. She wasn't sleeping well, uncomfortable no matter how she tried to lie, and had lost weight, a combination of a disinterest in food, and difficulty in keeping anything down. I reached out a hand in sympathy, trying to offer at least the reassurance that, come tomorrow, she would have a plan. At that, Indie returned with a *jebena* full of hot *kawa,* and three small, chipped, *sini* cups, and sat on the low wooden stool to pour it. In an attempt to dispel Selamawit's frustration, conversation turned to lighter things, and before long Indie was regaling her with the story of three of our newly hatched chicks who, somehow, managed to fall into the long drop, leaving Dawit with the unenviable task of attempting to scoop them out. As Selamawit wiped tears of laughter from her cheeks, Indie paused to deliver the final chapter of the escapade, which saw the chicks, just moments after Dawit had rescued them, turning around and falling straight back in. Pleased to see my friend laughing again, I sat back, smiling, a hand moving to my own bump as my baby danced inside.

Kawa finished, the card games lost by us all with accusations of far too much cheating all around to declare a fair winner, and dusk moving in, it was time to say farewell. Selamawit and I, already with plans in place to meet tomorrow so I could go with her to the hospital, stood waiting at the wooden gate that led into my compound while Indie collected her washing, hanging dry now in the sunshine, and put it away in the bag she kept at mine. Together, they walked along the dusty path criss-crossing the wide square of grass in front my house, turning to wave before rounding the corner and finding *bajaj* to take them away, Selamawit to the rooms she and her husband have in the staff accommodation at the government health centre at Darche, and Indie to the hospital.

The next morning, having been given a day off from my duties at Amorameda, I could have a rare few hours of rest. After serving Dawit *kawa* and breakfast, and holding open the corrugated metal sheeting that makes up our gate so he could push out the motorbike given to him by the Bishop in Emdibir for his journey to and from work, I turned back to the solitude of an empty house. I hadn't slept well, my baby determined to keep me awake with his movements, and looked forward to lowering myself back on to the foam mattress, pulling the cool sheet over my head, and sleeping. A couple of hours later, judging by the how the shadows had moved across the room, I woke once more. The room had warmed up with the day, mud walls ineffective against the effects of corrugated metal roofing that has spent hours in the sun. We needed rain, but weren't due any for a month yet, at least. And, actually, as hot and dry as the air was, with the *tef* harvest not yet finished, a downpour now would be disastrous. The huge mounds of *tef* need time to dry out, and the zebu, attached to wooden sledges that thresh the seeds from the stalks, need time to walk in their endless circles while the young men throw armfuls of separated crop onto the waiting *gare*, donkey carts.

Banking the fire, having just finished warming *kawa*, I heard the muezzin from the mosque in the distance calling out, summoning the worshippers for their lunchtime *dhuhr* prayers. It was later than I had expected. Selamawit would be waiting for me soon.

An hour later, sitting side-by-side on the examination couch, listening to Dr Rita explain the options for Selamawit now, I felt her shift beside me. She turned briefly to catch my eye, raising an eyebrow in question. I nodded with reassurance, and watched as she gave her answer to Dr Rita.

'Yes, I understand.'

'Good. So we'll go ahead with the miso?'

'Yes.'

With that, Dr Rita stood, and reached into the pocket of her white coat, hung over the back of the door that had been pushed half-closed for privacy. Outside, the voices of those waiting to be seen filtered in. There were people everywhere, waiting on benches outside the outpatient rooms, walking between the laboratory and the toilets, supporting relatives with arms in slings, carrying coughing children. Nurses in white coats weaved their way between them, trying to bring some order, ensure patients were seen in time. The place hummed with movement. But, with many years working here as a midwife, Dr Rita had asked the room be kept empty for Selamawit's consultation, so it was calm and quiet. Usually, four or five women were seen simultaneously, sitting opposite the midwives and surgeons carrying out the consultations at desks standing perpendicular to one another. Having found the small plastic pot that stored the pills of misoprostol, the drug used to start an induction of labour, Dr Rita motioned for Selamawit to open her mouth, and placed a quarter of one, 25mg, under her tongue. Selamawit grimaced at the chalky taste, and reached out to take the blue folder containing her medical notes that Dr Rita held towards her.

'Go to Delivery, give your notes to whoever is in charge. I think it's Indie today. I'm leaving in an hour or so, for a meeting in Addis Ababa, so I won't be here tonight, but I'll make sure Admasu checks in on you, and you'll have Indie and Atsede.'

Selamawit nodded, and I reached for the door, leading us through the crowds and down the slight slope to the green metal gates that separated the outpatients' departments from the hospital itself, smiling at the two huge tortoises that spent their days eating through the grassy patch kept just for them, delighting the hospital's youngest patients and their parents, alike. Calling out greetings to the staff as we passed along the veranda, Selamawit and I made our way slowly to the Delivery Room, catching site of the hospital cats dozing in the sunshine bathing the small courtyards that ran parallel to the wards, worn out, no doubt, from spending the night chasing the rats away. Overhead, huge blue and green butterflies danced between the flowers. Astroemeria, Indie had told me in delight one day, her favourite. The hospital was beautiful, with greenery grown over the decades by the Sisters taking up every possible patch of land. 'Never underestimate the power of nature in calming the soul and healing the mind', Dr Rita had told the gardeners, when they asked why they were squeezing yet more plants into the small space between the operating rooms and the surgical wards.

Pushing through the heavy wooden doors leading to the Delivery Room, I called out a greeting to Zekiya, standing bent over, explaining to a smiling young woman how to make sure her baby is latched on properly. She looked up and raised a hand in greeting, gesturing through the curtain that separated off the midwives' work area from the beds of the ward. We made our way through, wondering where Indie was, before coming across her crouching by the cupboard that held the medicine most often used in the Delivery Room, from antibiotics to analgesics, and those needed in cases of emergency: magnesium sulphate to treat pre-eclampsia, tranexamic acid for bleeding, adrenaline in cases of maternal collapse. She had a tatty notebook balanced, open, over one knee, and was counting out vials with a pen, then recording the numbers in the columns laid out. As Selamawit entered ahead of me, she looked up and smiled.

'Selamawit! Peace. You're here. Great. Have you seen Dr Rita? What's the plan?'

As she passed on her medical notes, Selamawit took Indie through the conversation with Dr Rita. Still listening, Indie took a few steps backwards, and leant through the door to put Selamawit's notes on the ever-changing pile on the desk, and scoop up a stethoscope, BP cuff, and pinard, the tools of a midwife. Returning to lean on the cupboard while Selamawit finished recounting the plan, she untangled the tubing of the BP cuff, and I moved to stand alongside her. Feeling Indie nudge me gently with an elbow, smiling and laying her hand gently on my bump, she turned, smiling to Selamawit.

'So, Dr Rita allowed this one to come with you, did she, Selamawit? I guess that means we can't get rid of her then.'

I narrowed my eyes and shoved her back, before taking Selamawit by the elbow and leading her to the chair next to the long, low cupboard that Indie had just been crouching in front of.

'Come on then, Sister Indie, get to work. Selamawit and I have things to do!'

Despite my teasing, 10 minutes later Indie had finished the initial checks for Selamawit and had reached out a hand to help her stand up before summoning me and leading us both to the door. She turned to face us and took both of Selamawit's hands in hers.

'Selamawit, everything is peaceful with your baby, and with you. So, now we try to help your body get things moving, okay? I know you're a midwife, and I know you've seen this a thousand times, but today, you are a mother having her baby. Don't think about anything else, that's what I'm here for. Walking, drinking, laughing, moving, climbing steps. They're all great. The bad news is, and I'm sorry about this, but you'll have to take Atsede with you. Who knows, she might be of some use fetching you water and mangos. Come back and see me in a couple of hours, unless anything changes in the meantime or you want to ask anything. This is exciting, Selamawit, we're going to meet your little baby soon!' With that, Indie released her hands and gave Selamawit a brief hug. Throwing a smile in my direction, she reached over and gave one of my braids a tug before spinning around and heading back to the midwives' desk.

'Okay, Selamawit, let's go.' The minutes ticked by as we started to walk. First, up and down the length of the hospital veranda, from the green gates near the tortoises down to the monkey trees providing shade for the benches of the Neonatal Unit. Then, when we could no longer bear to look at the same formation of tiles under our feet, we moved instead to the gravel path that stretches the length of the back of the hospital, dividing the compound between it and the church. The huge fir trees lining the walkway kept out the last of the sunset light, and as real darkness fell, we reluctantly found the concrete steps that would lead us back past the administration rooms and to the small staff café. Sitting, resting, and talking quietly, Selamawit suddenly leaned forward, caught unaware as the powerful muscles of her uterus tightened once more. After it passed, she leant back on her hands, breathing heavily. I murmured reassurances, and passed her the open bottle of water that I had been carrying, encouraging sips every now and then. We sat for a little while longer as Selamawit continued to contract, me continuing to pass her water. Our conversation, which until now had been lively, had quietened, with Selamawit concentrating on her breathing. As the minutes between the contractions shortened, the nausea set in, and not even water would stay down. Standing up, I moved to where I could see the clock in the staff café, and started timing Selamawit's contractions. Realising we had been walking for hours, I reached over to touch her shoulder and suggested we make our way back to Delivery, where Indie could listen in to the baby and make sure they were coping okay with the pressure of Selamawit's uterus bunching up around them. Nodding as the most recent contraction loosened its grip, I helped her to stand, and slowly we made our way back across the cobbles, pausing every few minutes, then down the slope, through the gates, and along the veranda, lit with the soft, glowing lights of the hurricane lanterns the night guards had placed at intervals along the walkway.

Indie was just where we'd left her all those hours earlier, eyes flicking between where her finger traced the writing in a file of medical notes, and the pen in her hand copying the details into a big book lying open in front of her. She looked up as we passed through the curtains and smiled, eyes assessing Selamawit intently before she turned to me.

'You haven't moved in hours, Indie! We've walked how far around the hospital, and you haven't moved.' I sat down, looking forward to resting my back, which had started to ache from so long walking, but somehow, all of a sudden, found myself on the floor, my gasp of surprise followed a heartbeat later by raucous laughter as Indie and Selamawit looked on. Deciding against Indie's help to stand up, given she still hand a hand over her mouth to hide her laughter, I looked more closely at the chair before trying again. Next to me, I saw Selamawit's hands tighten on the edge of the desk, and turned to Indie, nodding in response to the question in her smile.

'Yes, it's started! She's been having moderate contractions every couple of minutes for the last half an hour'.

As far as I thought, it wasn't necessary, at this stage, to do an internal assessment, to see whether Selamawit's cervix had started to dilate, and I hoped Indie would agree. Over the first few hours, or longer, of labour, the effort of contractions isn't necessarily to open the cervix. There is so much else going on, a transforming dance of the woman and baby, to prepare for the final moments of birth. Not only do the contractions have to alter the very anatomy of the cervix, encouraging the rigid muscles that have kept the integrity of the uterine cavity safe to soften, relax, and stretch up to become part of the lower segment, but also to guide the baby's head into an optimal position, to finish the job of loosening the ligaments and muscles of the pelvis, which started months ago with the changing hormone levels of the woman's body, and to give the woman time to adjust to her expectations of how it will feel. Only once all of that has happened can the contractions start their work in earnest, inexorably pulling the cervix open, and, little by little, pushing the baby ever downwards. I had a feeling that Selamawit was a little way from this point yet, and when Indie knelt at Selamawit's side, rather than asking her to lie on the bed, I knew she thought so too.

'Ishi, Selamawit, we've got a few minutes until your next contraction so listen. Everything is great, your baby is happy, Atse says you're happy, so the best thing now, as you know, is to keep walking. I'm not going to suggest an internal assessment yet, because its clear things are happening, and there's no need to interfere with that. You're doing great. This is the start, let's keep it going. Have you got a drink? Good, little sips then, okay?' Indie was talking softly, twirling the pinard in her hand. With that, Selamawit leaned to one side, resting her head on her shoulder, and breathed her way through another contraction. I yawned and stretched, grateful that I had the chance to sleep this morning, then reached out a hand to Selamawit. Once more, we started walking. It was cold and, beyond the small pools of lights from the lanterns, very dark, with the clouds gathering overhead not letting through any of the light from the moon or stars. The hospital was quiet, too. Evening visitors had left, and the night staff, having finished the medicine rounds, were no doubt settled into seats, weaving mats for the *jebena* pots, or embroidering *meskel*, cross, designs onto clothing. And outside, we walked. It was a much slower pace than earlier, with the length of each contraction longer, and the space between them shorter. We spoke quietly sometimes, but I could see Selamawit was happy to let the quiet of night settle over us as she breathed, and, after endless footsteps, started to groan through the contractions. I sat on the hard wooden bench, leaning back to rest, wondering if my baby was surprised to feel me still awake, or walked alongside her as the hours passed. Needing to rest for a few minutes, Selamawit led the way back to the Delivery Room, and to the couch where I had placed her plastic bag earlier. At least here, between the contractions, she could rest, lying on her side, one hand flung over her head, the other gripping the bars that held the mattress in place. Indie came by every so often, gently lifting Selamawit's long red dress just enough to press the wooden end of the pinard against her bump, smiling each time, hearing the baby's heart thumping. When I first started to notice tiny beads of sweat forming at Selamawit's hair line, and across the bridge of her nose, I quietly called out to Indie. With the next contraction coming, Selamawit somehow pulled her exhausted body into a sitting position, before pushing up onto her feet so she could stand and sway through the peak of it. Indie's face, pale in dim lights powered by the backup generator, appeared around the curtains, looking curious and eager. I smiled, and shushed her, nodding to Selamawit, whose groans had deepened to the sounds only heard from women coming to the end of their labour.

Suddenly, she stood upright, and a gush of amniotic fluid spread across the floor. I felt my eyes widen; there was a lot. It reminded me of my eldest sister, whose eighth and final baby, Beza, was born into my hands four years ago at this very bedside, also with a diagnosis of polyhydramnios. She had been breech, at least until my sister's membranes had ruptured, and as the fluid had spilled out over the floor, she'd turned at the last minute, an unexpected benefit of muscles loosened by seven previous births, to be born head first after all. I had laughed in surprise as my hands went to her head, her shoulders, her buttocks, guiding her out and to the waiting arms of my sister. Watching the spreading puddle at our feet, it seemed more now than I remembered at Beza's birth. Not as much as one woman from Dakuna who also came to mind, whose name I don't remember but whose waters filled emesis basin after emesis basin, and who must have had close to six litres of fluid, five times what you'd expect to see. Her abdomen had visibly shrunk as I felt the waters flow out between my fingers and over the palm of my hand, which I kept in place to ensure the baby's cord didn't get caught up in the sudden movement of water and prolapse through her cervix. She had gone on to have a beautiful boy, I remembered, despite the amazing amounts of fluid.

With her waters broken, Selamawit's groans changed again, as her body took over and instinctively began to push. Indie had retreated after seeing Selamawit's membranes rupture, but returned a moment later with the aluminium tin that contained clamps and scissors, and a pair of gloves. I stood, holding Selamawit's hands, waiting for Indie to prepare, but turned around when I felt her hand on my arm. She held out the gloves and smiled at us.

'It should be you, Atse. I've already asked Zekiya, she doesn't mind, and I'm sure that's what you want, isn't it, Selamawit?' The contraction fading, Selamawit nodded, and once more allowed herself to fall gently onto the bed. I took the gloves and pulled them on. I could see the tell-tale bulging and stretching of her tissues that indicated her baby was moving through the birth canal. There was no need for internal assessments now: in just a few short contractions, the baby would be here. 'Selamawit, your baby is coming soon. Do you want to stand? Crouch?' A shake of her head.

'You can stay on the bed if you want. Indie will get more pillows, then you can sit up a little?' A nod this time, as Indie reached through the curtains to the next bed, thankfully unoccupied, and brought another of the pillows to prop under Selamawit's back and head. 'Better?' Another nod. 'Okay, follow your body. If you need to push, push. You're ready, I'm ready.'

Trying not to disturb Selamawit's focus, I gestured to Indie to open the tin, so I could reach the episiotomy scissors I needed to help the baby navigate her perineal tissue, distorted by the thickened scars of her circumcision. They wouldn't soften like the perineum itself. 'Selamawit, I need to open you a little, with an episiotomy. I will only do it when you are pushing, and the baby's head is right here. But don't be afraid if you feel the scissors beforehand. Okay?' She grimaced but nodded, having said just the same to thousands of women in her role as a midwife. Indie had said that in England, women don't have episiotomies often, and if they do, it's nearly always after the anaesthetising effects of lidocaine have numbed the area. We didn't have enough lidocaine here to give it to all women birthing – it was kept instead for the serious injuries that needed suturing in the Emergency Room – so episiotomies were performed and repaired relying on just the fortitude of the women to get through the pain. That was one thing we were both determined to change at our Clinic, and with the scissors in place, I wished we had already opened so that I could give it to Selamawit now. Another contraction, and the head of Selamawit's baby came down to push against the back of my gloved fingers. It was time. Waiting until I could see her contraction peaking, I felt the scissors cut through her skin, giving the baby space, and when I felt it was enough, quickly slipped them back out and onto the tray before using both hands to catch her baby as she came out all at once.

Smiling and sighing happily, I passed the baby up and onto Selamawit's chest, where Indie was ready with a towel to place over them both, my eyes still on the fabric underneath her, which, I had noticed, was already drenched with bright red blood. Had it been some minutes later, I would have expected this, likely a result of the separation of the placenta. But that was unlikely to have happened yet, and giving the cord a gentle tug, I could feel it wasn't ready to come. Where was the bleeding coming from then, I wondered? It wasn't the episiotomy site either, for when I placed a gauze over that, blood continued to seep. My mind ran through the possibilities. Perhaps she'd had a tear higher up, that wasn't immediately obvious. Had there been a slight abruption, a result of the polyhydramnios, and this was the blood that had remained trapped inside until the baby was delivered? Concentrating on this, I hadn't noticed that Indie had left until I looked up to ask her for another set of gloves. But now I saw she wasn't there, and I realised the baby wasn't either, and then the silence struck me. Selamawit had her eyes closed, her head to one side, and her hands resting on her chest. She was whispering a prayer. I recognised the rhythm of her words even if I couldn't make them out exactly. Where were the cries of a newborn, with lungs adjusting to breathing air for the first time?

When I heard Indie's voice call out for Zekiya, I felt as if I had stepped into the rain, and a wave of cold fear hit me. My head snapped in her direction.

'Indie, is everything okay?' I had forced my voice to stay calm, but I could hear the waver.

'Oh, God.' It was Zekiya. My hands trembling, I looked back to Selamawit's bleeding, which, actually, had slowed a little. Knowing that my responsibility was Selamawit now, and that Zekiya and Indie would take of the baby, I tried to drag my mind back to her, and started speaking.

'Selamawit, Indie and Zekiya are with your baby now, *ishi*. I'm not sure why they thought she needed more help, but they are both there, and they will take care of her. You were bleeding a little, but it seems to have settled down. I'm going to repair the episiotomy, and then see if I can help them. But you were so brave, *anbessa*, lioness, and I'm sure Indie and Zekiya will look after your baby.' I couldn't think of anything else to say, but kept repeating that her baby was being looked after and that I would go and help as soon as I could. I tried to close down the part of my mind that was resolutely three metres away, with Indie and Zekiya at the neonatal resuscitation area, desperately listening for a cry, and instead focus on doing my best for Selamawit.

When I'd finished suturing, and was content that her bleeding was no more than usual, I pulled off my gloves, and went to stand at her side. 'Selamawit, I'm going to go and see your baby now, okay? I'll make sure someone comes to tell you everything. I'm sorry I don't know more, but I'm certain they're doing their best.' Selamawit turned her head to look at me, tears in her eyes, but she nodded and squeezed my hand.

'Thank you, Atse. I'm so happy it was you here with me.' Selamawit can't have seen how guilty I felt, or she wouldn't have said that. I smiled weakly, searching for the right words.

'I'll always be here with you, Selamawit, you know that. Let me go and see what's happening. Are you cold? Come onto your side, I'll get you a blanket.' Changing the bloodied white cloth under her, I glanced to the resuscitation area, my eyes finding the backs of Indie and Zekiya, working side-by-side, quietly talking to each other. I couldn't see anything of the baby, but from the way Zekiya's shoulders were moving, I knew she was still doing chest compressions. How many minutes had it been? All the time I was suturing, and talking with Selamawit, and now standing here. Then I realised, what was I doing just standing here? Grabbing a thick woollen blanket from the cupboard, I quickly threw it over Selamawit, making sure she was covered, before resting a hand on her arm for a brief moment

'I'll come back as soon as I know, honestly. Selamawit... I ...' I didn't know what to say, instead turning away, and making my way across the room to Indie and Zekiya. It felt like every step was a huge effort, as if I were walking through a river, not air. I desperately wanted to know what had happened, but at the same time was so afraid of what I would see. Taking a deep breath, I stepped up next to Indie. Whatever it was I had been expecting, looking down at my friend's daughter, it was not this. When Indie took the mask from her face, to see if there was any change, any attempt to breathe, I felt the fear wash over me. How could this baby survive? But how could Selamawit if she didn't? I'd seen so many different babies during my time as a midwife, but I'd never ever imagined this. What had happened deep inside the genes and cells of this baby to see her born without a nose? I looked to Indie and Zekiya, concentrating on counting and continuing with the resuscitation. Performing the rhythmic, methodical chest compressions, even on a body as tiny as Selamawit's daughter's, was tiring, and I could see the tension across Zekiya's arms. Pulling on a pair of gloves, I gestured my intention to take over, unable to speak. Zekiya nodded with relief, and as Indie gave the puffs of air, trying to keep the baby's lungs rising and falling and her blood full of oxygen, she stepped away, half turning as if to make her way to Selamawit before stopping and raising her eyes to me helplessly. I understood. She wanted to go to her, to say something, but didn't know what, or how.

'Zekiya, it's okay. Stay here, help Indie keep count. I'll talk to Selamawit, after...' As I said it, I felt Indie and Zekiya turn to me, the same thoughts passing over all three of us. After what? I didn't finish, my eyes flicking back to my hands, resting on the fragile bones of the baby's ribcage, waiting for Indie to finish. Two, three. After the third puff of air, it was my turn. Thirty compressions. I felt her tiny body as I pressed down, immensely grateful for her soft bones that shouldn't yet need to break for my attempts to be successful. I wanted to pray, but I couldn't bring any order or coherence to my thoughts. I heard Zekiya start to count in Guraginya, and concentrated on the cadence of the numbers, somehow calmed by knowing that she was counting in our language. *At, hwet, sost, arbat...* When I heard her reach thirty, I stopped, and Indie took over. *At, hewt, sost.* Back and forth we went, passing the heavy responsibility of bringing Selamawit's baby back from the edge between us. Time warped in those minutes, with nothing to give any meaning to time except Zekiya's chanting voice. *At, hwet, sost.* And then I thought I felt a heartbeat under my fingers. Weak, but there. And then, our own breath held in a mixture of utter disbelief and overwhelming relief, as we watched, her chest rose and fell. She gasped. Against all the odds, despite all our fear, she gasped. Watching Selamawit's baby come back to life was a moment I will never forget. It felt like flying. A weightless, floating moment of respite from fear. Knowing that we couldn't stop now, not until her breathing was established, Indie and I kept going, with Zekiya's counting now tinged with hope. When her arms started to move, and she drew her legs up to her body, colour flooding her ashen skin, I couldn't believe it. This was after. She was alive. Selamawit's baby was alive. Next to me, Zekiya stopped counting, and sat back. On my other side, Indie remained silent, staring at the baby with tears in her eyes. I felt it now, the ache in the muscles of my hands and forearms, and flexed my fingers, trying to loosen the tightness, wondering if it would work on the aches and tightness of my heart too.

Selamawit's baby slowly opened her eyes, blinking, her clenched fist waving randomly at her side, the uncontrolled movements of a newborn testing each part of their body. The question in my mind now, of course, was where do we go from here? I turned to Indie, wondering if she had any more idea than I did. But when I caught her eye, I saw the same mixture of relief and uncertainty that must have been in my own. And when Indie's hand knocked against the tiny glass vial secured carefully with a small length of surgical tape to the side of the tray holding the resuscitation equipment, I knew her thoughts echoed mine too. Do we give her this? Are there other, unknown differences deep within her body that might react to the mechanism of Vitamin K, given to prevent bleeding? I had no answers, and no idea. But worse than that, we were alone. Was it really just this afternoon that I had been standing in the doorway, listening to Dr Rita say she was travelling to Addis?

Thinking back, what happened over the next few hours is hazy. I remember the moment when the baby stopped crying and she also stopped breathing. I remember talking to Selamawit, trying to explain, to give some answer. I remember Indie's starfish, and, minutes later, Dr Toni's voice constricting as she said we had to get the baby to Addis Ababa for further investigations. I remember how the relief I had felt at her breathing slowly faded to be replaced with doubt. A doubt that still lingers today. Liyu is almost four, now. She's just learnt to smile, which has been the greatest gift she could have given to Selamawit after so long without any indication that she recognised her mother at all. Like Indie, I feel responsible for this remarkable girl, and her even more remarkable parents. And every time she contracts pneumonia, which is often, I am afraid we won't be able to guide her through it. But, somehow, we do. Which is as much a testament to the enduring, limitless love of Selamawit and her husband Kibru for Liyu as any medical or clinical treatment. I have never felt so humbled by the power of a mother's feelings, nor so proud, as I did watching Selamawit breastfeed her baby, taking her off every few seconds so she could breathe, then reattaching her. Having breastfed two newborns now, and felt the discomfort those first weeks, I am as in awe of her today as I have ever been. By all reason, Liyu shouldn't have survived the transition between womb and world, nor the weeks in the hospital in Addis Ababa, nor the bouts of illness that saw her gasping for breath. But, somehow, she has. And when she reaches five years old, the doctors from America told us a little over a year ago when we travelled to meet them, maybe there will be surgical, or medical, ways of helping her to do so.

Having a child so different from everyone around them is difficult everywhere, but here, where there is no help, no access to physiotherapists, speech therapists, dieticians, occupational therapists, specialist education services, no wheelchairs, it is almost impossible. I wonder, sometimes, whether we would have continued the resuscitation for so long if she hadn't been Selamawit's daughter. I wonder what life we condemned her to. But then I watch her smile at Selamawit, and I watch Selamawit smile at her, and I have to believe that our actions that night were meaningful.

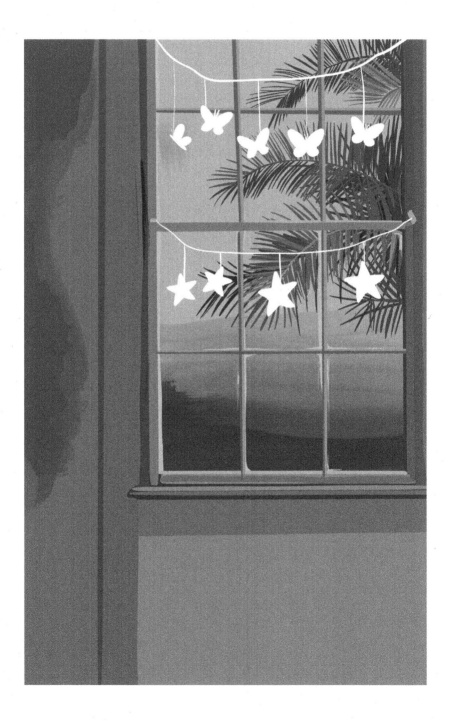

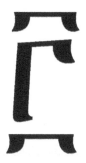

3

Mahaza

Indie

'Good afternoon, Adi.'

'Are you a doctor?' Her dark eyes narrowed as she asked. I could feel the suspicion rolling off her in waves, tinged with something akin to anger. She would have been beautiful when she was younger, and was still a striking figure now, braced in the doorway, feet planted firmly and arms crossed protectively across her chest. Her long red dress was tied at the waist with a blue scarf, with tassels that almost reached her knees and moved hypnotically as she shifted. Bound around her hair was a matching blue scarf, and glittering at her ears, neck, wrists, and fingers was beaten, tarnished silver. As the *sheyhr's* wife, she was powerful in her own right, and almost more feared than him. 'Are you a doctor?'

'I am a midwife.'

'And did your mother also care for women?'

'My father's mother'.

She regarded me with narrowed eyes, calculating something, but what, I wasn't sure.

'That is enough, come in'.

I risked a glance sideways at Atsede, unwilling to show my own apprehension, but needing reassurance. Her eyes were cast down as a mark of respect, but her stance was easy, relaxed. I breathed a sigh of relief, happy to have been considered enough, and followed Adi through the door into the darkened room. We were offered stools at the long, low table that stretched the length of the small room. A plastic flower in a Coke bottle sat on the polished wood, next to it a chipped jug of water and an upside-down metal cup. It was hot, and the walk across the open meadows to get here had left us with a sheen of sweat across our faces and arms. Before entering the compound, as we had looked at each other to arrange scarves and hair, and beat off the thick red dust kicked up as we walked, Atsede had laughed, as she always did, at my pink cheeks. A gift from the sun. Now I could feel the cool depths of the hut, a welcome relief. While the corrugated iron roofs are sought after as a mark of prosperity and progress, the traditional thatching, held up high by a thick central pole, often a full tree trunk with knots and branch stubs still attached, is far more effective at keeping out the heat of the day.

'Atse?' I whispered, aware that we could hear movement behind the curtains dividing the single room in two.

'Mm?'

'Why did she ask if I was a doctor?'

'She doesn't trust them. She thinks they've forgotten the old ways, forgotten how to treat people, rather than just diseases. They are too enamoured with their big machines and small pills.'

'And midwives?'

'Oh, midwives can't help but remember. It's woven into our heartbeat.'

I liked that, and sat a little straighter. We had come to see her daughter's daughter, a little dot of a baby born just a day ago at home. The pregnancy and birth had been straightforward enough, but the family were worried now, saying there was something strange coming out of her, pushing against her skin. It was at the same time vague enough and specific enough to be alarming, so after opening up the Clinic's doors, sweeping out the accumulated debris from the night patients, and greeting the day staff, we had squashed into one of the ubiquitous *bajaj* tuktuks and made our way through the town, already bustling with fruit and vegetable merchants, the herders with their zebu, and students making their way between lectures. Hurtling at an unlikely speed between them all were the *bajaj*, with scant regard for any sort of safety, and yet daintily side-stepping almost certain disaster on an hourly basis.

Joining us in the back were two older women, woven baskets deftly swung from their backs onto their laps, and a couple of chickens bound at the legs with *enset* fibres tucked between their feet on the floor. With four in the back, one person had to shift sideways, to sit half on the seat and half on the jerrycan eased into the tiny space. With two more people joining the driver in the front, both clinging on to the metal struts of the roof in order to keep their balance, the *bajaj* was deemed full enough to see us right the way through the crossroads and along the three kilometres of bumpy, dusty track to the referral hospital. Beyond this, up the gulley, across the meadows, and through the forest, lay the first of the villages that spread out across the mountain tops. This was Atsede's home. After extricating ourselves from the *bajaj*, and handing over a few tattered notes, we set off down the rocky slope to the dried stream bed at the bottom, laughing and chatting as we went, calling out greetings to the shopkeepers that lined the way and to nurses on their lunch breaks sitting in the cool shade of the avocado trees. At the bottom of the slope, the well-trodden path branched off. Left led, after a while, to Atsede's family compound, where her mother, aunts, uncles, and several cousins still lived. A while further, along the path we would be taking, were more huts, more families. At the end of that was the *sheyhr*. To the right, by the river, was the house of the village's chief, and a few huts down, Selam's family. Surrounding them all, and filling in the spaces, were hundreds upon hundreds of trees, plants, and flowers, beehives, zebu, chickens, and monkeys. It was a place teeming with life. Even in the arid months without rain, when the river ran dry and the blue skies stretched on forever, in the shade beneath it all, fingers dug a few inches into the soft ground came up damp. It wasn't this way for many other parts of Ethiopia, suffering through devastating drought, but the mountains were protective, allowing the land to retain some moisture even in the driest months.

Walking, with knee-high tef waving gently in the breeze, we had the rare chance to spend uninterrupted minutes together, time to go through our days at the Clinic without supplies to stock or medication to check or notes to write or clients to see. It had been busy over the last few weeks, with women, surrounded by women, coming to birth their first, or third, or fifth, baby. Patients, too, had come, seeking treatment for malaria, pneumonia, or typhoid, for burns and cuts and rashes. Atsede had started to teach me part of the botanical lore she had learnt as a young girl, which herbs and leaves to find for teas and tinctures. Distracted by our musings, we covered ground quickly, and before long saw the wooden fence that ran the length of the *sheyhr's* compound. Rounding the corner, grateful that the end of our sun-drenched walk was near, we had straightened our clothes, and prepared to knock on the door.

Now, the sound of rustlings behind the curtain materialised into the shape of a small bundle appearing, preceding the *sheyhr's* wife. It was the baby we had come to see, sleeping peacefully, one hand resting against her forehead, the other no doubt nestled close to her side.

'Give her to me.' Atsede suggested gently, reaching out to taker her.

The blankets twitched slightly as the baby startled with the movement, and her eyes snapped open. After hours of staying in the darkened world behind the curtains, the sunlight streaming in through the open door was the first time she'd been aware of such brightness.

'Shh, Mimi, it's okay. We're going to look after you.' Atsede was watching with tenderness as the little girl stretched, and opened her mouth to protest. With practiced ease, Atsede unwrapped the tiny baby, deftly lifting her hat to feel the fontanelles, where the bones of the skull, yet to mesh together and harden into one continuous arch protecting the brain, are still forming at this young age, with a soft spot in the middle that reacts to significant illness by either bulging outwards with infection or sinking inwards with dehydration. Satisfied that there was no indication of anything serious there, Atsede continued her examination, talking all the while to the baby in a soft, lilting murmur. As Atsede moved down her little body, placing a hand over her chest to feel her breathing and heart, the baby once again scrunched up her eyes as her mouth popped open to sound her displeasure. Atsede took the opportunity to put the end of a finger in, checking for the suck reflex, feeling the roof of her mouth for a hidden cleft, her gums for teeth. When the baby started to suck instead of cry, Atsede left her finger there, and motioned instead for me to continue. Lifting up the cloth that had been tied around her waist to serve as a nappy, we saw straight away why we had been summoned. It was not, as we had feared, an omphalocele, caused when the skin of the abdomen fails to meet across the middle and around the umbilical cord, leaving intestines or, in the worst cases, the liver and other organs, protected only by a thin, see-through membrane. Smiling at each other and the *sheyhr's* wife in reassurance, we let out sighs of relief. It was an umbilical hernia, marked to be sure, but fairly common, especially in babies born prematurely, which this one looked to be.

'She is beautiful, Adi', Atsede began, 'she looks like her grandfather!' It was true, even so young, a shadow of the *sheyhr's* distinctive smile could be seen on the lips of the baby, and her eyes, just a little more widely spaced than her mother's, echoed his in shape.

'And on her stomach? What is that?' Adi's tightly controlled expression relaxed when looking at her granddaughter, the first child of her first child, and the slight tremor of her hands gave away her fears for the baby.

'It is called a hernia', I explained, 'And you don't need to be worried. Most of the time, it will go down by itself, and it will be as if it was never there.'

The sound of shouting voices came from behind the curtains, and suddenly, tumbling through, were the boisterous sons of the *sheyhr's* youngest brother, jostling and laughing. It was a welcome distraction from the intense scrutiny of Adi, who couldn't keep watching us while also chastising the boys for their interruption. Smiling and waving at Atsede, and nodding to me with a little more apprehension, they managed to contain their laughter and play long enough to apologise before Adi shepherded them out like errant goats. I turned to Atsede, grinning.

'Adi, like Indie has told you, there is nothing to worry about for now. We want to you to keep an eye on it, and make sure it isn't getting any bigger, and also make sure the baby doesn't show any signs of becoming sick, like a fever, or refusing to breastfeed. But otherwise, we will come again in three months to check on her. You know you are to take her to the hospital for her vaccinations?'

Adi nodded curtly, no doubt not taking kindly to being told what to do. But Atsede's reputation and standing in the community protected her. There weren't many women Adi would take direction from.

I gathered my courage to speak again, 'Adi, could we see your daughter? I want to congratulate her on such a beautiful child.' It wasn't entirely true, and I could see Atsede trying not to smile as she started to rewrap the baby. She was beautiful, in the way all new babies are, and congratulations were certainly in order, but it was more that I still wasn't comfortable with clinical information not being given directly to the baby's parents, regardless of who the grandparents were. It had got me into awkward positions before, inadvertently causing a chief from another village to be quite affronted when I asked to talk to his daughter instead. I had learnt enough from this to know not to approach the situation so openly, but I was still a midwife, and I still had a duty to the baby's mother. Adi narrowed her eyes shrewdly, fully aware of what had happened in the past, before beckoning us through.

The baby still in her arms, Atsede stood up next to me, and we made our way around the table, and passed through the curtains into the warm, dark, quiet world of the *chyne*, the postnatal period. Taking up her position on a wooden *burchama* stool beside her daughter, Adi stayed to chaperone. Talking quietly – anything else seemed out of place in this place of shadows – we sat and listened to Adi's daughter tell us of the birth, as is the custom, before offering our compliments. At that, Adi stood to escort us out, with Atsede following suit, raising her voice a little to ask a question of Adi about the zebu in the yard, fussing just a fraction longer than necessary to get her *netela* scarf in place. I took the chance, and leant over to whisper quickly about the hernia, telling the new mother not to worry, but to keep an eye on it, and that we would come back soon, and that her daughter was beautiful.

Eyes blinking against the sunlit room, in bright contrast to the dimness within that we had just become accustomed to, Atsede and I turned, smiling, to thank Adi for her hospitality before making our way to the door, and then, with less subdued steps, across the grass of the compound and out to the freedom of the fields, where we laughed, delighted at our small deception, and how well our meeting with Adi had gone. The walk back along the paths worn by the countless footsteps of people and lifestock passed quickly, especially after Atsede reached into her bag and produced a small bunch of bananas and a couple of mangoes that would serve as lunch. It was early afternoon when we handed over a few *birr* to the *bajaj* driver, and stepped back through the blue metal gates of the Clinic, just in time to meet the first women arriving for their antenatal check-ups.

'Indie!' Atsede's voice sung out through the sunshine, and she walked lightly along the veranda, turned the corner, and looked into the Laboratory, elbows propped on the wooden windowsill, smiling. 'Having fun?'

I was not having fun. Having chosen the hand without the stone when presented with Atsede's clenched fists held out in front of her as we sat in the *bajaj*, I had spent the rest of the afternoon dipping urine, checking for infection markers, for protein, for sugar, for ketones, the repetitive task broken only to record results on the slips of paper passed through the window by women with apologetic smiles handing over small pots wrapped in bits of tissue. Meanwhile, from a room ringing with laughter and voices, Atsede had been seeing the women who come to us for care throughout their pregnancies, feeling for the lie of their babies, listening to the beats of tiny hearts. Sulking, I threw the used dipstick into the red bucket that serves as an infectious waste bin with flourish and turned away pointedly, more to hide the smile I couldn't stop than anything. On top of it all, I also had the hiccups.

Laughing, Atsede threw the petals from a flower she'd had in her hand at me. 'It's your fault you're here, Indie, you chose the wrong hand. Anyway, it's been me the past two clinics, so it's only time. Stop being so dramatic.'

'That is not hygienic, Atsede Kidane.' Hiccup. 'We can't have plant waste all over our laboratory!'

'Best clean it up then, hadn't you?' I narrowed my eyes in response as she continued. 'And it's hardly plant waste, they're petals!' Hiccup. '*Ere*, Indie, who is thinking of you! Raphael.' Pause. 'Mesmora.' Pause. Hiccup. 'Diego.' Pause. 'Your mother, your father.' Pause. Hiccup. 'Selam… Aha! Selam.' She was listing the people in my life important to me. At Selam, my hiccups stopped. 'It's Selam, then! When did you last see her?' Shrugging, I smiled, still holding my breath. 'Well, those who think of us like to be thought of in return, like those who love us like to be loved in return. At least your hiccups have stopped now you've remembered her! So, will you listen to me? Get your white coat, you've got a patient.'

Laughing, I obeyed her command. I loved her Gurage explanation for hiccups, that someone is thinking of you, and the solution of naming the one responsible for the thoughts, thus thinking of them in return, is certainly more straightforward, and far less likely to end in wet clothes, than drinking a glass of water upside down.

Delighted to get out of the four white walls of the laboratory, and away from the pots of urine and recording ledgers, I let Atsede take me by the hand and lead me to the Emergency Room. Inside, sitting on the green plastic chair next to the desk and wrapped in a thick white *gabi,* despite the heat of the summer, was a tiny, stooped figure, with a heavily wrinkled face, and solemn eyes looking out from underneath a hat pulled down low over her forehead. Next to her, sitting tall and statuesque, was a striking young woman, wearing a flowing green dress with a yellow scarf bound around her hair. It had golden thread woven through it, and golden disks dangling from the edging that caught the sun and sent a sparkling light over the ceilings. The two could not have been a greater contrast in pictures of health, yet the way their smile lit up their faces as we entered was identical. Atsede and I took our places, me at the desk ready to take notes, and Atsede perched on the brightly patterned Malawian *chitenge* cloth that covers the examination couch when not in use.

'*Enate*, what brings you here? What's the matter?' I spoke in Amharic first, almost certain these women weren't from the villages. The dark blue tattoos etched across the chin and neck of the older woman, and on the forehead of the younger, were far more commonly seen among the Tigray people from far to the north of the country. When the response came in Amharic, heavily inflected with the sounds of the Tingrinya language, my suspicions were confirmed. The younger woman, the granddaughter of our patient and the only one of the two who understood Amharic, answered, telling of the struggles her grandmother had been having, the weaknesses, the confusion, the light-headedness, how her voice had become quieter, and her walking more difficult. Atsede smiled gently, letting her finish before offering advice. She had called me because she knew of my fondness for the elderly men and women who came to the Clinic, amazed by their lives and all they'd seen, but of the two of us, she was the nurse, and far better placed to give advice. I was there to assist, really, and write the notes. As Atsede spoke, I took the blood pressure cuff and wrapped it around the papery skin of the older woman's upper arm, careful not to catch her with the harsh velcro. I started to pump the small black bulb, tightening the strip of fabric, but stopped almost at once. Her blood pressure, I knew straight away, was far lower than we'd expect, less than half of what it should be. I unwrapped the cuff, took the stethoscope from my ears, and turned to Atsede, hesitating to interrupt, but concerned.

'Atse, it's very low. Maybe we need to see about her going to the hospital.'

I could see Atsede thinking something through. She opened her mouth as if to speak but closed it again, several times, clearly trying to find the right way to start. Then, with a voice I've only heard her use with children, she started to speak to the women. Pausing often to find the right words, wanting to be both kind but also honest, Atsede explained. This grandmother, great-grandmother actually, who had seen so much in her long life, was now an old woman. The systems within her body that had worked so hard to keep everything stable over the previous decades were, as Atsede phrased it, simply tired. And as they became more tired, they couldn't work as effectively. Eventually, they wouldn't work at all.

'We can send her to the hospital. They can put needles in her arms, medicine into her veins. But it won't heal her, it will only mask the underlying reality. Your grandmother is old, soon she will die.'

I felt myself wince at Atsede's words, but couldn't deny the truth of them. And as her granddaughter translated the words, it was clear that is what the old woman had mostly been expecting to hear.

'If your grandmother is in pain, we can help you manage that.

If she has difficulty breathing, that too we can help with. But the best thing you can do with her is to take her home. Keep her warm, keep her comfortable, keep her company, and keep her loved. Just be with her. Make the most of this time.'

The conversation went back and forth between the three of them for some time, but I stayed mostly quiet, uncertain of what to say. When a natural lull in questions came, Atsede brought the consultation to a close and the young woman stood, guiding her grandmother into the waiting *bajaj*. Before the woman had a chance to be bundled in, she turned to us, and spoke in Tigrinya. Neither Atsede nor I understand the language, but the lilt and cadence of her words echoed those of the Guraginya blessings, and the tender tone of her voice wasn't lost on us. As she finished, she inclined her head in thanks, and smiled once again, her eyes all but disappearing among the deep wrinkles. It was an infectious smile, and we couldn't help but return it, moved by her gratitude.

'Atse, why didn't we refer her? They can manage low blood pressure.' I was puzzled. The old woman hadn't seemed sick, and certainly hadn't seemed like she was close to death, and yet Atsede hadn't recommended treatment.

'Indie, you come from a culture afraid of death, willing to take extraordinary steps to keep it away. We aren't the same here. When people grow old, they die. When people are very sick, they die. That's just how it is. This isn't a reason to be scared. It's just another part of life. It's just letting go, and trusting in something more than what we can see, in God. Think about it for a while… as you get back to the laboratory and all your urine!' It was a gift of Atsede's to mix profound lessons on faith and fate and life and death with the lighter realities of matters at hand. It was her way of keeping things in perspective, to not get too caught up in the existential questions that, inevitably, come with a profession so caught up in the extraordinary moments of birth. 'I'm not playing, Indie, go on! We've still got at least 10 women to see.'

Atsede finished with an affectionate laugh, an understanding look in her eyes, and a hand resting on my shoulder for a moment, before turning and, sweeping up the waiting women in her wake, leading the way into the Maternal and Child Health Room. Shaking my head at her retreating figure, I stood for a moment with the old woman's notes, encased in a blue paper folder with her medical record number written across the front in big black font, in my hands, then sighed, added them to the pile on the desk, and made my way back to the Laboratory, my mind full of what Atsede had said.

The sun was just starting to sink below the horizon when we finished for the day, pulling closed the wooden shutters against the cold night air, and locking up the rooms unlikely to be used overnight. Raphael and Mesmora had already made their way back to the house, laughing and gambolling together like puppies, accompanied, as always, by Yordannos. Ever grateful for the Ethiopian schooling system, which only sees pupils attending for half a day, allowing the rest of the time to be spent helping around the house, in the fields, with the livestock, or, as with Yordannos, playing with the younger children, Atsede had chivvied them along an hour or so earlier, not wanting them to be caught in the coming rain. I wasn't sure her plan would work, though, knowing full well the three of them were likely, at this very moment, to be clambering up and down the huge pile of mud that had been dumped just outside the house, to be used, eventually, to make the new kitchen; our current one, having suffered through one too many rainy seasons, was crumbling around one corner. For now, though, it was an adventure playground, providing hours of amusement for the neighbourhood children, who took it in turns to scramble up and then fling themselves down. Our sons may have been among the youngest of the group of children who spent their afternoons roaming the tracks and trails, chasing goats and climbing up the wooden fences, but Yordannos kept an eye on them, and they had soon learnt to join in, often returning to the house as dusk was falling, tired but happy, with leaves in their hair, scrapes on their knees, and smiles on their faces. It was an idyllic childhood for them. Smiling at the thought, a sudden cracking sound caught my attention.

Desu, the guard, was splitting wood for the fire that would keep him warm through the night. It was an ongoing mystery where his constant supplies of wood came from, it being something of a treat in this part of town, far from the river and the trees it waters. Usually, firewood is bought from one of the merchants who brings it in by donkey cart, or collected by children sent to the forest in the afternoon, and yet, within a few minutes of arriving in the evening, Desu strolled back into the compound with an armful of wood. We suspected he may have been taking bits and pieces from half-finished fences that had been put up haphazardly to demarcate plots of land, but we were never quite brave enough to ask him about it, not being entirely sure what we would do if it turned out to be true. The thudding of the axe had taken over from the afternoon chorus of the small red and blue sun birds that danced through our trees and the coo of doves nesting in the rafters over the veranda, and almost covered the tentative knocking on the gates of the Clinic, pulled mostly closed to stop the wild dogs coming in during the twilight hours.

I caught sight of the movement of a familiar figure, bent double, hands clasped around the bars, and heard the tell-tale groaning of a woman in labour. It had just started to rain, and the skies overhead suddenly seemed much darker than they had a few minutes ago. While we had sat in the last few hours of sunshine that day, the big black clouds had been amassing on the horizon, and there was static in the air, along with the oppressive feeling of a storm on the way.

'About time,' Desu had said as the rain started to fall, 'this has been coming all week'. He was right; it had been sticky and humid for days now, and even the long, loose dresses worn here did little to keep sweating bodies cool.

'Mahaza!' I called out, 'We're here, open the gates, get in'. The rain was coming heavier now, and the first distant rumbles of thunder could be heard. Lightning flashed suddenly, and Desu appeared from the guard's room with a big umbrella to guide Mahaza into the Birth Room.

Opening the doors of the big cupboard that took up much of the back wall of the room, I shifted aside the piles of beautiful green elephant-patterned newborn clothes donated to the Clinic, to find a blanket. Straightening up as the most recent contraction released its grip, Mahaza took it gratefully, wrapping it over her thin shoulders.

'Mahaza, your baby certainly knows how to pick a night to be born! How are you? When did your labour start?' The door creaked, and we both looked over as Atsede slipped in, pulling it closed behind her.

'The storm is definitely here. Mahaza! What a night.'

Laughing, she gestured to me. 'That's exactly what Indie said.' Her smile faded as her hand went to her stomach. 'Ah, you'd have thought I'd remember from the last one, but I never do. These *cortat* are painful!'

Atsede and I exchanged glances, smiling in sympathy. This was Mahaza's sixth baby, and with all five of her previous babies born into Atsede's waiting hands, there was never any question in Mahaza's mind that she would walk the paths to the Clinic this time as well, despite the distance and the darkness. Mahaza's breathing deepened as the contraction reached its peak, and she moved her head from side to side, eyes closed, teeth bared in a grimace. As this one passed, Mahaza shook her head, 'Atsede, you tell me now, six is enough!'

'Ah, I'm not sure. Indie, what do you think?' She looked at me, winking.

'I've always thought eight or ten a perfectly good number of children.'

'*Besmahah!*' Mahaza exclaimed in mock horror, crossing herself, 'In God's name, eight or ten! No. This is it for me.'

Laughing, Atsede shoved her gently. 'I seem to remember you saying exactly that last time! And yet here we are, once again.'

'Mmm. But I mean it this time.' Her minutes of respite between contractions coming to an end, Atsede motioned Mahaza on to the mat on the floor, where she could feel through the skin and muscles to map out the lie of Mahaza's last baby. I sat down at the desk, lifting the registration folders out of the way to find the rosewood pinard that I had used since first becoming a midwife. Finally seeing it, tucked behind the vase of silk flowers kept on the desk, I turned just in time to watch as Mahaza moved onto her side, a familiar expression creeping over her face. Atsede sat back on her heels, a hand still resting on Mahaza. She looked over to me, mouthing 'still breech'. I nodded in acknowledgement, not troubled that this baby would be coming feet first, but running through how best to help Mahaza.

Pushing herself off the floor, Atsede joined me at the desk, pulling a stool out from underneath it. 'You'll take the lead, okay?' I smiled gratefully at her, feeling, as I often do, so privileged to be under her guidance. Breech births aren't considered particularly unusual here, and certainly no emergency, but as they are not as common as vertex presentations, there wasn't often the chance to keep up-to-date with skills. With Atsede watching quietly from the corner, this would be a good opportunity.

The night deepened and darkened around us, with rain continuing to pour from the sky. Atsede's husband had called an hour or so ago, to let us know that the boys were curled up under blankets with Yordannos, the three of them jumbled together blissfully unaware of the storm raging. They had, exactly as I had imagined, played outside on the mud until the *zinab*, the rain, started in earnest. With bellies full of scrambled eggs and avocado, a favourite of Yordannos, they had blinked sleepily before Dawit had pulled out blankets from the trunk and thrown them over their warm little bodies, asleep almost from the moment they lay down. A few kilometres away, in the birth room, Mahaza continued to groan as her contractions increased in strength and frequency.

Atsede and I were taking it in turns to walk with Mahaza, rubbing her back or holding a glass bottle of sugary Mirinda while she took small sips. Looking around, a sense of contentment stole over me. This was the experience Atsede and I had wanted to give women. The soft glow of the fairy lights strung up around the room bathed us in a gentle light, so at odds with the gusting winds and crashing thunder outside. To keep the mosquitoes at bay, we had lit incense in the four corners, thin streams of scented smoke curling in the air. It was, above all, peaceful, and so different from the harsh spotlights and cold corners of the Delivery Room at the hospital.

We knew it was unlikely to be that much longer: after five births,

Mahaza's body remembered how to move a baby through. As her groans deepened, becoming more primal, more involuntary, Atsede stepped back, nodding at me to step forward. Mahaza, mostly, had been walking, or resting between contractions on her side on the mat on the floor. As she started to bear down, she squatted, taking her into an optimal position for allowing her pelvis to shift just enough to allow her baby through. Sitting just behind her I watched as she stretched and opened, little testicles arriving first. I smiled at the indignity for the poor baby, and his introduction to the world testicle first, then glanced up at Atsede, just in time to catch her controlling her own smile. My concentration back on Mahaza, more and more of her son appeared with the next contraction until, at its peak, his legs, bent at the knee, were released. I had been waiting for this, and reached out to gently support them, keeping my hands just beneath his buttocks. Had it been a first or second baby, Atsede would now be reminding me to support the baby's body across my forearm, and remain vigilant for signs that it was time to help, to turn the baby a little so his head would descend more easily with the last stages of the birth. With Mahaza, though, I had expected this not to be necessary, a suspicion confirmed looking at Atsede, who held up her own hand in a 'leave it alone' motion. She was talking quietly to Mahaza now, reassuring her to push as she needed. In an awkward position half lying on the floor behind her, I willed the next contraction. As soon as I thought it, I watched as the baby's arms were born, falling to his side as they did so, followed a heartbeat later by his head. Thankful that my hands were there already, ready to scoop him up as he slipped into them, I smiled in delight and relief. Mahaza knelt forward onto all fours, resting muscles aching from having held the squat through such an intense time. Her baby, already wiggling in my hands, opened his mouth to protest as I passed him through her legs and up into her waiting arms. As I had come to expect when breech babies born to women with several children already are given the time and space to make their way out, it had been calm and controlled. No shouting doctors, no emergency bells, no stirrups or episiotomies.

The spluttering cry of a baby clearing his lungs for the first time, an action which results in a complete change in how his body is oxygenated, starting the closure of the vessels bringing blood from the placenta and instead utilising the oxygen in the air as, for the first time in nine months, he breathes, had just started when it was muffled as Mahaza expertly manoeuvred her nipple into his mouth. Mahaza had her eyes closed, her head resting to one side. Atsede smiled at me. *Well done,* she mouthed, wrapping the thick blanket over Mahaza and her son. I grinned back, *thank you.*

'*Enkuan des alesh,* congratulations on your happiness, Mahaza.' Opening an eye, Mahaza smiled wearily at me, her arms full of her new son. Even through the blanket, I could hear the slightly frantic snuffling of a baby trying to find the nipple.

'Well, that wasn't so bad after all.' She was watching her baby, one hand shifting to cup her breast and deftly move him to it. In front of us, Atsede laughed.

'It isn't over yet, Mahaza! Let's see about getting this placenta delivered, and then get you two settled down. It's late, and raining, you'll stay here for the rest of the night, with us.'

It was a little over an hour later that Atsede helped Mahaza onto the bed as I finished mopping the floors and wiping down the equipment. The clamps and scissors used on the umbilical cord were submerged in a bleach solution, ready to be cleaned and sterilised in the morning.

The delivery of Mahaza's placenta had been straightforward, with no concerning bleeding afterwards. Desu had a fire going in the steel firepit, one that he kept fed all night, a big pot of water boiling, and the clay *jebena* balanced in the flames beside it. The hot water was for Mahaza, a shower to wash away the fluids of birth, before pulling on a fresh dress and woollen cardigan, and then hot *kawa* for all of us. Yawning and stretching, wishing each other *wahay worit,* good sleeping, we took our places for the rest of the night, Desu on his chair at the fireside, Mahaza and her son warmly tucked away with blankets on the bed, and Atsede and I under the twinkle of the fairy lights on the floor.

We were lying flat on our backs on a thick mat made from the fibres of the *enset* tree roots, our shoulders pressed close together so that the coarse woollen blankets would cover us both. Now the night was even colder and completely black, a deep, endless darkness broken only by flashes of lightning dancing across the sky. Once again, above us the thunder rumbled, so close and so loud I could feel my bones trembling. Quietly, I shifted onto my side, turning to Atsede. A cold eddy of air crept in under the blanket before I could tuck it in, and I heard an involuntary gasp from Atsede. The lighting flashed again, and I could see it reflected in Atsede's eyes as she smiled reassuringly.

'I've always thought that there's something so ancient about thunder,' I whisper, not wanting to wake Mahaza or her baby, 'it's so timeless, so unchanged, so far beyond our control.'

'Does that scare you?' A rustle of blankets, another gust of cold air, as Atsede also turns. Facing each other, only able to make out each other's features when the sky was alight, it feels as if we are the only two awake in the world.

'No, not really. It just makes me realise we are only here for such a brief moment in time. And think about all the lives that came before us, and all the ones that will come after.'

Again the rumble of thunder, and Atse glanced across the room to check that it hadn't woken Mahaza before replying. 'I worked it out once. If you imagine your mother, and your mother's mother, and her mother, going back over 500 years, and then the same for your father, well there were more than five thousand. All for us to exist in this moment in time. Can you believe that? We are only here because five thousand of our ancestors were here first.'

We were quiet for a few moments, both imagining the intricate web of lives that had somehow convened in us, lying here on the floor of our Clinic in the middle of the night, in the middle of a storm. Then Atsede continued, trying to find the words. 'Each of them must have loved, and lost, and wept, and laughed. How many stories did they have to tell? How many times in their lives were they faced with triumph? With disaster? How many were midwives, like us? Would they be proud of us, do you think?'

Lost in thought, I listened to Mahaza's quiet snoring. The even quieter whimper of her new son could just about be heard through the thunder. What a night to be born, I thought once again, in the midst of such a wild storm. What a night to witness a birth. Atsede spoke up again, in the mood to talk.

'We call it *borja*, the lightning, and everyone is a little afraid.'

'Of the lightning?'

'Yes, definitely. *Borja* brings fire and, if it chooses, death.'

I felt a shiver travel the length of my spine at her whispered words, and looked out through a crack in the shutters to the night sky, not sure what I was expecting to see, before turning back to Atsede.

'Are you scared, Atse?' I reach out a hand to take hers in reassurance, just in case. She squeezes back with gratitude and continues to talk in quiet tones.

'In the village, during the last *berga*, *borja* chose a *sahrbet* to burn. Within minutes, it wasn't so much a fire as an inferno. Everything was lost. Just the central pole was left, a black, charred, crumbling stump.'

'And the family?' I almost didn't ask, didn't want to hear the answer, vividly remembering the blistering skin and hollowed eyes of the two young children who barely survived another *sahrbet* fire, set by their mother in a moment of psychosis. The brittle thatch and zebu dung walls burnt hot and fast in *berga*, the dry season, with smoke and flames filling the space in a matter of moments, drawn upwards into the eves of the pointed roof.

'For some reason *borja* didn't take anyone, thank God. One of the younger sons was struck though, when he ran outside. Don't you remember? He was on the Children's Ward at Attat.'

I did remember. The brother, Lemma, was alright, amazingly, except for the burns that spread across his torso and abdomen, and even these weren't painful, he said. I had joined the surgeons on their rounds that morning, mostly to greet the women recovering from caesarean sections performed during the night, or the day before, but also because I enjoyed the experience, the camaraderie. My first thought on seeing Lemma was that his burns were beautiful. The current of electricity that struck him had followed the superficial branching of tiny veins usually invisible just under the surface of the skin, burning them black, so now it looked as if a fern had been tattooed over his body. He was in good spirits, with a raffish smile, and confessed to enjoying the attention his unusual injuries brought, deliberately leaving his t-shirt off, and his sheet pulled back so he couldn't be missed. The vitality and liveliness of the youngster was welcome in the Children's Ward, where so many are so sick and so sad.

Often full, with two patients to a bed, and more on mats on the floor, the Children's Ward opened its doors to patients suffering from a huge variety of diseases, some needing weeks of medication, some just a day or two. It was a steep learning curve for the student nurses and recent graduates to be placed here, and there was much to learn, not least just seeing how fast children become unwell, but also how fast they recover.

Sharing a bed with Lemma was another, younger boy, whose mother was trying to bring down a soaring temperature with cloth soaked in cold water then pressed against his body. Having stayed to chat with Lemma, I was now several cases behind the surgeons, who had made their way through the narrow gaps between beds and around the low wall that divided the room in half. I wondered about hurrying to catch up, but as I glanced once more at the woman bent over the bright yellow bucket of water, I realised it was Birkenesh, a relative of Selam's, and instead stayed to help.

Like the children themselves, their immune systems are young, and still learning. This means they also have a tendency to overreact to even mild infections, unsure how dangerous they'll be and so wanting just to get rid of them. This is why fevers in childhood are so common: they are the immune system's way of trying to kill off the invading cells. The problem is, an immune system going haywire can also end up damaging healthy, normal cells, leading to more significant problems than the initial infection would have. It's a balancing act. For some diseases, like the itchy chicken pox, the defence mechanism of a child's response is actually better than that of an adult. There aren't many, but there are some. Malaria, on the other hand, is not, and it was for this that Birkenesh's son was receiving treatment. I would often find Selam at his bedside over the week to come, and it was a joyful day when I first noticed she hadn't disappeared for hours to help cool a fever and calm a sad, scared child. Birkenesh's son recovered well, with the remarkable stamina of youth and a fierce drive to survive. Lemma, too, had been discharged, happy to be going home but devastated, he had confessed to Birkenesh and Selam, that his lightning marks had faded until they were almost invisible.

'No one will believe me now!' he had lamented, forgetting of course, that almost everyone in the village had been to see him during his stay on the wards, not to mention the fact that his hut had burnt down. Able to laugh again now her son's malaria was under control, Birkenesh and Selam had teased him endlessly.

'Ask Indie to print the photograph off! Then you can keep it with you all the time.'

'Good idea. I can even sew it onto your forehead, if you wanted. That way everyone will see it!'

Laughing, the women had kissed a blushing Lemma on the cheek and helped him wash his hands and face before waving farewell as he took the hand of his older sister, and started the walk home.

A sigh from Mahaza as she changed position bought my attention back to the present. In the distance a hyena whooped, followed by the harsh bray of a donkey, keen to avoid a confrontation but not afraid to kick out in defence if one ventured too close. Glancing at the silhouette of the window, the flickering quality of the light told me that Desu had, more than likely, just added another log to the fire, flames rising higher around it. I pushed myself into a sitting position, looking over at Mahaza. I could just see her hand, draped protectively over her son tucked in at her side, exposed to the cold night air. She didn't seem to mind though, and neither she nor the baby had woken. Settling back down on my side, I saw Atsede's eyes were closed now, and I wondered if she was sleeping. A wave of tiredness crept over me and, yawning, I pulled the blanket up under my chin and gave in to sleep, my last thoughts those of gratitude for nights like these, my son cared for with love and laughter by his young friends, allowing me to be guided by women like Atsede to take part in the most ancient ritual of all, birth.

Atsede

'Good afternoon, Adi.'

Indie had spoken first. I could tell from the way she held herself, her hands twisting nervously around the length of her *nutella*, and her carefully controlled Amharic, that she was nervous. I smiled to myself, taking the blame for her apprehension as, over the years, I had told her many tales about the *sheyhr*. As a child, I grew up frightened of his other-worldly power, but as an adult this was tempered with a better understanding that the influence he held was a result not of the intervention of the divine, but rather of the faith put in him by those to whom he offered guidance. The *sheyhr*'s wife, on the other hand, was fierce enough even before considering her connections to the occult. But we had been asked to come, and regardless of her stern countenance, I knew she was glad we were there. I moved slightly closer to Indie, leaning against her for a moment in reassurance, glancing up briefly to see the *sheyhr*'s wife with her eyes narrowed, poised to speak, before looking back at the hard-packed mud floors, indented with decades of footprints, wondering what we would find inside.

While Indie held her own under the scrutiny of the *sheyhr*'s wife, I thought more about our days at the Clinic over the last few weeks. It had been busy, the rooms full of movement and voices. Several days, also, with the sounds of new life, and one memorable night when I had barely a chance to pull on the blue gloves before a baby slipped easily into my hands on the tiles of the veranda. Indie, having stayed at our house for a few minutes after I started the walk to the Clinic to settle our sons into the care of the young women who lived with us so they were able to attend the schools, had missed it altogether. She only arrived after I had passed the little baby up to the breast of his mother, who wrapped her arms and her blanket tight around him and smiled happily, and guided them into the protected warmth of the room, lit with flickering candles in the absence of electricity. She had clapped her hands delightedly at the unexpected speed of the birth, and laughed at the shellshocked look on Lemlem's husband's face. It is still very unusual for men to be present through a birth, and instead the women gather around, lending quiet, unobtrusive support.

As I sat, watching Lemlem helping the baby nestle to nurse while we waited for the delivery of her placenta, my mind wandered back to the birth of my nephew. My sister and I had worn a track through the dusty gathering space in front of the Catholic church that shares grounds with the hospital. In just one moment, she had turned to me, complaining of a twinging cramp, and before we had a moment to register, her son's head was crowning, and a heartbeat later I had dropped to my knees to prevent him landing in the dust. The shock rendered us speechless, both staring wide-eyed at the baby in my hands, before I gathered myself enough to call out to the guards keeping watch from the balcony. Hana, our cousin and a midwife at the hospital, appeared a few minutes later, panting from the run and bearing armfuls of towels. Together, we helped my sister back to the Delivery Room, where clean clothes were waiting for her and her child. Only after she was settled into the warmth of a blanket tucked over her and the baby, did we realise what had happened, and laugh until tears streamed over our cheeks. It was as much from relief as amusement. From there, I let my memory of my own labour come, walking endless steps through the mango trees, willing the contractions to start, laughing at Indie's attempts to encourage me into what she called lunges, a feat I found quite impossible given that the swell of my bump meant I could hardly keep my balance on two feet planted firmly together, never mind apart. Despite Indie's best efforts, my contractions never started, and in the end my tiny son was born following the intervention of Dr Rita's faithful scalpel. And, of course, there was Indie's birth, the hours and hours of contractions, through the evening, the night, and the next day. She hadn't wanted much, just water sometimes, and the hum of talking in the background so she knew she wasn't alone. I will never forget how, as Alem and I talked quietly, sitting on the floor of her room as Indie leant against the wall, we had jumped at the sudden slap of a hand on the wall.

'Bimbi. Mosquitoes.' Indie had said by way of explanation, smiling ruefully before the next contraction took her breath away.

After a decade of midwifery, I am still struck, every time, by how different each experience of birth is, but before I had too much more time to muse on this, I was roused from my memories by a lull in the conversation between Indie and the *sheyhr*'s wife. I shook my head as I came back to the present moment, and gathered, from the gesture of the *sheyhr*'s wife through the open door of the *sahrbet* hut, that whatever Indie had said was enough. She had passed the unknown test. Following her into the strange atmosphere of a dim hut after the bright sunshine, my mind was still very much on birth as we sat on hard, three-legged stools, and waited to be told what to do next.

'Atse?' It was Indie, turning to me as she reached out to straighten the flowers on the table. 'Why did she ask if I was a doctor?'

The *sheyhr* knew about healing, of that I had no doubt. While many others offer questionable advice, sometimes even dangerous, I have long respected this *sheyhr* for his willingness to work alongside the clinicians of the area. His wife, on the other hand, remained quite suspicious of doctors, disliking the desk and gloves and white gown that separated them from those seeking treatment. Midwives, though, did not cause her to prickle in quite the same way. We lay our bare hands on the women in our care, skin on skin, and become their confidantes, developing a relationship spanning their childbearing years and beyond. We feel the history of the midwives who have gone before us, continue many of their superstitions, uphold many of their beliefs, practise many of their ways. For this reason, the *sheyhr*'s wife accepted us in a way she never would the doctors.

We waited for a few moments longer, listening to the muffled, muted voices coming from behind the curtain stretched across the doorway dividing the hut in half. In many of the *sahrbet* huts, these areas were reserved for the zebu cows and their calves, a place to keep them safe from the dangers of the night. It was this way in the huts of my family, and more often than not the doleful eyes and flopping ears of a black and white face could be seen appearing around the corner of the dividing wooden wall, searching for leftover squares of the pounded *enset* root dough biscuits, *wussa*. Their gentle lowing lulled my sisters and me to sleep too many nights to remember. The *sheyhr* though was rich enough for the zebu to have their own space, leaving the hut for the sole use of the family. Just as I was about to ask Indie where the cows live in England, the *sheyhr*'s wife reappeared, holding a bundle of blankets tenderly. I motioned for the baby, but felt just a moment's hesitation before Adi handed her over. This was the first daughter of her first daughter, and though she was little more than few handfuls of hours old, she had clearly already won over her fearsome grandmother's heart.

As soon as I took the baby into my arms, I could see why. She was beautiful, with dark, smooth skin, and even darker eyes, the shape the same as those of the *sheyhr*. Lying her on my lap as Indie moved the stool closer to help, I started to move the blankets away, starting with the soft, tight curls of her hair, and making my way down to her abdomen, where a small curl of her umbilical cord still lay, tied off with twine made from the fibres of the *enset*, a certain indication that she was born at home. It looked clean, though, and I wasn't concerned. When Indie's hands reached across to help move away the cloth gathered up between her legs and tied around her waist, we saw the reason we were here at all. A fairly large umbilical hernia protruded out just under the umbilicus. I heard Indie breathe a sigh of relief, and murmured a prayer of gratitude that this little baby would not suffer through the difficulties of an omphalocele.

I smiled reassuringly at Adi as Indie and I explained what we had found, but as Indie spoke up once more, it became a smile of conspiration. Indie had, for the most part, adapted easily to the ways of life here in the Gurage mountains. But some things she still struggled with, and this was one such example. The *sheyhr*'s wife, as the matriarch of the family, would accept our advice and guidance for the care of the baby, without us needing necessarily to tell the baby's mother, particularly given her position of respect in the community. But Indie couldn't quite accept this, and had, once before, already slighted the chief with her wish to talk directly to the mother of the patient in question. It wasn't a significant enough infraction to cause real offence, and her open, ingenuous approach to the situation was her saving grace, but I knew she was being more careful this time. I was proud of her for this, for trying to fit into our ways without compromising her own sense of duty. She must have seemed convincing enough to Adi, although I could hear the unspoken intention behind her request to offer her congratulations to the new mother on her beautiful baby. Still, it was a small deception, and I intended to play my role in allowing her to have a few moments of privacy with Adi's daughter. When the time came to take our leave, I suddenly found myself unable to untangle my *nutela* from the strap of the bag that contained the tools of midwifery, and paused in the entranceway to the curtained-off area, blocking Adi's view of the bed, where Indie briefly crouched.

Indie's jovial steps as she came through the curtain to join us told me all I needed to know about whether or not she had had the time to talk to Adi's daughter. Smiling at our own cleverness, we bade farewell to Adi, and started out along the worn path through the waist-high grasses swaying in the breeze, following the well-trodden path back to the road, and back to the bustle of noise and life and activity awaiting us at the Clinic. The sun overhead was higher than I expected; we had been gone the whole morning. Looking further towards the horizon, I groaned quietly at the dark clouds just starting to gather. More rain, then. It was just as well I had remembered the mangoes and bananas in my bag as we walked back through the *meda*, the grasslands, as those would have to do for lunch. It was inevitable that this afternoon, the time for antenatal appointments, would be busy.

I heard the *bajaj* pull up to the blue Clinic gates before my name was called. Judging from the exuberant beats of the music playing, this wasn't an emergency. When it is, the *bajaj* are silent.

'Kokeb, everything is at peace with your baby, there are no problems. We're just waiting for your urine results, Indie's doing that now, but your baby is in the right position, his heartbeat is strong, and he is growing well. Is there anything else you want to ask?' Kokeb shook her head, smiling easily as she turned onto her side before sitting up, legs swinging slightly as she sat on the side of the examination couch. 'And you remember what we've talked about? Try and rest when you can these last few weeks, and make sure that little one is moving around, okay? If you have any problems, we are here. You have my phone number, just call.'

I smiled as Kokeb thanked me, pulled her dress back into place, and left, pausing briefly to talk with the women sitting on the benches outside. She would deliver nicely, I was sure, looking forward to the day she came to us ready for birth. I stood too, stretching away the aches of an afternoon sitting and bending over pregnant women, an ear to their bellies, or a hand on their chest. In college, we were taught to use thermometers, but I trust my hands more. I was tired, but happy. Many women had come to us this afternoon, in all stages of their pregnancy. Some you wouldn't even know they had a child on the way, while others came with the unique walk of the heavily pregnant, body tipped back slightly to make up for their growing bump, with steps moving from side to side as much as forward, hands clasped at the breastbone, resting on the swell of their unborn child. While I loved being there for the moment of birth, there is something special about seeing women in their pregnancy. So much hope and happiness, all centred on an entirely new soul. There was a change in the hum of conversation that came in through the window as the women all spoke at once to tell the *bajaj* driver where to take the patient he had brought. I heard several call his name, along with questions about his health, and that of his young daughter, and recognised it as belonging to one of the drivers usually around this area, whose own wife had pushed her baby into Indie's hands not so long ago. As I finished writing Kokeb's notes, I could hear the women cooing outside. He must have shown them a photograph of the baby. I caught his eye as I made my way to the Emergency Room, pausing to scoop a jug of rainwater from the *roto*, the barrels used to collect it, and scrubbing my hands with the disinfectant soap.

'Showing off your baby again, Fele?' Feleke laughed, turning to me with his hands raised in guilt before handing over his phone. 'Oh,' I sighed, 'He is sweet! Is this from his christening?'

'Yes! Doesn't he look handsome?' I smiled and nodded in

agreement, before passing his phone back and continuing along the veranda. Just a few steps ahead of me, already inside the room, were two figures, one standing tall and straight, the other much smaller, but so bundled up in a *gabi* it was difficult to discern much at all. The taller, her dress floating around her, and the disks on the *shajsh* bound around her hair clinking musically, helped her companion into a chair, then turned to greet me.

Taking my place in the blue chair at the desk, I offered my greetings as I took in the two women in front of me. The *gabi*-shrouded figure was a tiny old woman, her face, the only part of her not tightly wrapped, heavily wrinkled, and around her temples wisps of white hair could be seen escaping the black scarf that seemed to be the unofficial uniform of the *shamagalet*, the old women. But for the dark tattoos on her face, marking her as Tigray, she reminded me of the elderly mother of my cousins, and I felt myself warm to her instantly. The younger woman, her daughter, or perhaps granddaughter, looking more closely, had beautiful peanut-coloured eyes which stood in contrast to her dark skin and which were, at the moment, clouded with concern. Looking again at her grandmother, my suspicions confirmed as she spoke, I could see why. I offered to bring Indie in for the consultation, knowing already what I would say, but also knowing that bringing in another clinician would provide the reassurance that her concerns were being taken seriously, even if no treatment was given. Explaining where I was going, I stood and made my way along the veranda.

Indie was engrossed in her task, and as much as she pretended to moan about being bored of the monotony, I knew she quite enjoyed being in the Laboratory, keeping everything in order and making sure the tests were all done properly. Not like at the hospitals, where the results are often made up. Her handwriting was neater than mine, too. I knew she'd heard my approach when I leant through the window only to be faced with her back. The pen dropped hastily onto the ledger, rather than being back in the pot alongside the strange collection of things that inevitably ended up there, everything from bandage scissors to a stick of sugarcane, gave her away, as did the fact she was now aimlessly looking at a blank wall. I couldn't help but laugh, and glanced down at my hands, at the petals I'd swept off the bench under the bottlebrush tree. Our eyes met as she turned, hers narrowing. But before anything could be said, I'd tossed them in and we watched as the bright red danced through the air, landing in her hair and on the paperwork. Laughing in earnest now, I reached for her hand, and we made our way into the sunshine.

Indie's eyes lit up as we entered the room, delighted, as she always is, to be seeing the *shamagalet*. As the granddaughter spoke, I heard the words I was expecting, the same words I had said not many years ago about my own grandmother when she, too, came to the end of a remarkable life. The low blood pressure reported by Indie confirmed this and I wondered how to say what needed to be said. That, yes, there were certain medications that could be given to mask the symptoms of a tired body coming to the end of its tenure on earth, but that, really, all the granddaughter and her family should do now was to be there with love. I remember being disappointed, initially, when I had been told this. I wanted the nurses and doctors to try everything to keep my beloved *agotey* alive, and couldn't understand why they were giving up so easily. But in the days that followed, I came to appreciate the gift they had given us. Instead of in a crowded, stressful hospital, with the daily sting of needles and chalky taste of pills, with strangers around us watching as we changed her clothes, *agotey* spent her last weeks propped up with pillows in the corner of the *sahbet*, with the soundtrack of her giggling grandchildren and great-grandchildren teasing clucking chickens and lowing cows, and warmed by the sunlight streaming in. She had hand-fed mouthfuls of *wot* and scrambled eggs, with endless cups of spicy *chai*, rich *kawa*, and cold *ihkha* brought to her by attentive daughters. Her friends and family spent hours at her side, reminiscing and remembering. She knew nothing but happiness in those days. And when she took her last breath, it was contentment that was in her eyes before they closed. She had had a good life, and a good death. I wanted that for the women, both the old one and the young one, sitting in front of me. Trying to find the words for all of this, I spoke slowly, carefully.

And while I could see resistance in the beautiful granddaughter, as she translated my Amharic into the Tigrinya of her grandmother, it seemed something akin to gratitude with which my words were met there. As I answered what I could about how the days were likely to pass now, Indie was quiet, listening.

She asked me, afterwards, why I hadn't suggested a referral, and I tried, once again, to explain that death isn't something to be frightened of. It isn't something that needs to be hidden away and only talked of in hushed voices. Whether you believe in Heaven or Paradise or nothing at all, as long as those who have died are thought of, something of them still lives on, and death isn't the end. I could see Indie needed to think about it, so sent her back to the cool, quiet Laboratory, where she would have time to herself. I watched her walk away, wondering if all *ferenji* were so afraid of what happens after life, then turned, smiling at the brightly-dressed women in front of me, ready to talk about birth instead of death. There was a spirited conversation happening, with much gesticulating and laughing. Kokeb hadn't gone home yet, I saw, and seemed at the centre of the mêlée.

'....and then, she gave her the *chura*! And you should have heard her scream. The *chura* wasn't even alive! "What am I supposed to do with this!" she said. "Well, give it to Indie, the *ferenji* eat them", the old woman had said, shoving it into Atsede's hands. Honestly, she nearly cried.' Laughter echoed down the veranda. Chiding Kokeb gently for telling the same story yet again, I couldn't help but smile too, remembering all too well the time I'd been tracked down on my walk back to the house from the market, and presented with a snake for Indie's lunch. It's a widely held belief that *ferenji*, foreigners, eat snakes. Unlike *habesha*, Ethiopians, who don't. When I'd handed a baffled Indie the stick with the snake dangling from it, she had laughed and laughed, then admitted that, while white people didn't often eat snakes, in a country called France they did eat *kandouta*, snails! We had spent a very entertaining evening comparing what is and isn't eaten, which also became a chance to continue Indie's education on the Gurage medicinal lore, like the healing qualities of the eggs of *jigera*, guinea fowl, and the meat of *jart*, porcupine, in relieving the symptoms of asthma, hunted only by the Funga, with their wickedly sharp *tor*.

Kokeb, having finished with her story, waved farewell and made her way out of the gates. Shaking my head at the still chuckling women, I took hold of the slightly older woman closest to me, Konjit, expecting her twelfth baby in the coming days, and steered her into the waiting room. I had known Konjit since I was a young child, living in Buchaj with my eldest sister, and was happy that she'd listened to my advice to slow down a little towards the end of this pregnancy. Usually, Konjit would be collecting firewood to sell at the market, instead of sitting in the sunshine talking with the expectant women.

'Konjit, how are you? How are you family? Your children? I am happy to see you here. Thank you for coming.' She smiled tiredly back at me, sitting heavily and fanning herself with the end of the scarf wrapped around her hair. It was an image so familiar to me, one I remembered from my childhood as Konjit's stomach swelled time and again with her sons and daughters. I remembered, with an unexpected wave of nostalgia, visiting her after a birth, only to be taken to one side by her daughter, the same age as me, and being told in a conspirational whisper than tonight was the night of our neighbour's *neprawr*, an esoteric ritual far more exciting than those that came with yet another new baby. A zebu bullock's skull, stripped of skin and muscle but with the huge horns still intact, would be propped up against the old tree and coated in spicy, clarified butter. Offerings of food would be left in front of it all through the night, accompanied by pleas and prayers, for good health and good harvest and good luck. Sneaking out with Konjit's daughter that night to see it was both exhilarating and frightening, as much for knowing the *awrie*, the wild animals, would come, attracted to the smells of food, as for not quite knowing what else was being summoned. The food our neighbours made, the special ceremonial dishes made for weddings, funerals, celebrations, would feed us all for days.

Konjit shifted in her seat, and I smiled. 'How is Nyana? I haven't seen her for too long. I miss her.'

'She sends love and peace, and did say she will come and see you. She will be with me when this one is born, God willing.' With that she gestured to her abdomen, rubbing a hand across it. We had spoken, at length, about whether or not the safest place for Konjit to birth would be at the Clinic or at the hospital. With so many previous births, there was a chance that the muscles of her uterus would not tighten up again after the birth, causing bleeding. As much as I wanted to be with Konjit as her baby came, I felt that perhaps this wasn't the best decision. Konjit had listened intently to my explanations before conceding that maybe the hospital would be better. Knowing that Nyana, who had trained as a midwife a little time after I had, and now worked in hospital far to the south, would make the journey to be with her mother during the birth was reassuring.

We had worked together briefly, years ago before Nyana had gone south, and I remembered now that our shifts always seemed to end in the strangest situations, like leaping into the back of a huge Izuzu truck, used most often to transport blocks of stone from the quarry, which had been put to work to transport a mother with no means of getting to the hospital, or turning around in the midst of cleaning cupboards to find another woman in a wheelchair being brought into the Delivery Room, the outline of her baby's body already visible through the fabric of her trousers. Nyana and I helped to peel them off, the baby's angry cries just about covering our surprised laughter at seeing the placenta, also delivered, flop onto Nyana's shoe.

As I moved my hands over Konjit's stomach, I was struck once again by the incomprehensible, incredible gift of pregnancy, of the unborn baby developing beneath my touch, exactly as it should, to be born in just a handful of months. It was difficult to believe it was once Nyana walking around this womb. Finding the baby's back, I reached for the doppler and turned it on, pressing a little deeper to find the thud of the baby's heart.

'Konjit, all is at peace with your baby. You have nothing to worry about. I think the next time I see you, this stomach will be empty, and these arms will be full! Have you thought any more about whether you will want another baby afterwards? Or what I said about maybe this one could be your last?' I didn't want her to feel forced into a decision, but I also knew that her body would be tired of being pregnant.

'Yes. I spoke to my husband, too, like you suggested. I think this will be my last baby. I would like the operation, like your Aklila.' I smiled at the mention of my oldest sister, and Konjit's oldest friend. They had known each other for decades, since Aklila had been courted by the young men, and Konjit, already married, had sat with her as our father chased away the families that came offering dowries. In my village, Aklila was known as the most beautiful, and most desirable, and it was a point of constant exasperation for my father, who wanted her to stay in school rather than marry. After months of proposals, and after my father had sent Aklila to stay with his brother, several hours' walk away, a journey she made one morning holding a letter from my father to my uncle explaining everything, Konjit had been there at the council held by my older cousins, giving Aklila the choice of what to do with her future. She had chosen Girma, and they had married that same week, settling down in the hut next to Konjit in a village an hour away. It was this village that I would move to some years later, to live with my sister and her young daughters. I spent almost 10 years there, under Aklila's the watchful, loving eye. As her daughters grew up, I taught them to make fire, to wash clothes, to cook. Every Sunday, after church, we would carry bundles of clothes and blankets to the river to be cleaned, before flinging ourselves into the fast-moving water. In exchange for their help washing clothes, I taught them to braid hair, allowing them to practise on me before styling theirs for the coming week. Konjit's daughters would be sitting next to us, washing their own clothes and braiding their own hair. The camaraderie and laughter lightened the work, made a game of exertion.

'*Ishi,* Konjit. I think that is a good decision for you. I'm finished here, you can go. If you aren't already *chyne* in two weeks, you can come again. But I don't think I'll see you. You have to keep resting now, Konjit, don't work too hard.' With that, I helped her up, and walked with her to the door, waving goodbye as she stepped off the tiles of the cool veranda and greeting the next woman, laughing as we realised we were wearing the same *shiti* dress.

The rest of the afternoon slipped by as women in all stages of their pregnancy passed through the doors. With the clouds still gathering in the distance, I called Yordannos from the game of stones she was trying to teach Mesmora and Raphael.

'Yorde, do you want to go home? The rain is coming. There are mangoes and bananas in the basket if you get hungry. And this,' I handed her a couple of coins fished from inside the drawer in front of me, 'is for avocados. Elsabet has some. Indie and I should be home, but in case we haven't finished here, there are eggs, too, for *erbat,* for the evening meal.' The young girl standing in front of me smiled and nodded, taking the coins from my palm, and encouraging the boys to their feet, suggested a race up the small hillock. I watched as they leapt from mound to mound, smiling to myself at Raphael, who had only just learnt to jump. As I watched, Mesmora lost his footing and fell over, only to be swept up a few moments later by Yordannos, laughing as she tried to swing him into the air. Raphael ran over to them, wanting to play too, and the three of them, pushing into each other, rounded the corner, following the well-worn path back to the house.

Looking further up the track I saw the familiar figure of Desu, the guard at the Clinic, walking towards us. I waved a hand in greeting, too far to shout one, and watched as he took the road to the Dom Boscan nun's house, no doubt to buy bread for the night. Trying to gauge the time, made ever more difficult by the sun's disappearance behind the looming clouds, I turned back into the Clinic, where the final two women of the day were still seated. I could hear the sounds of evening at the Clinic: mops being swished over tiles, Indie and Alem sweeping away the dried mud with small, handheld brooms made from the stalks of stiff grass, bound with string of *enset* fibre. Alem had sat with Indie one afternoon a few days ago, teaching her how to twist and twine the tough white strands. The *macha,* the brooms, they were using now were the result of these lessons, and so far seemed to be holding up, a fact that Indie liked to keep reminding me of after I teased her for her string not being tight enough.

As I ushered the last woman in ahead of me, I heard the gravelly voice of Desu calling out a greeting. Sure enough, in one hand was a small round of bread and in the other a jar of honey, no doubt harvested that afternoon. It was the time for honey, our own hives at home filling the air with the distinctive, sweet scent of full combs. Alem had come to meet him, passing over the keys and the solar-powered torch that had spent the day precariously balanced on the branches of a tree charging, high enough up that neither the boys nor the goats could reach the strap dangling so temptingly, and pull it down. We'd learnt that lesson quicky.

As I glanced at the yellow-bound maternity notes in my hand, checking that they did belong to Tsega, I saw the white sticker. HIV hasn't ravaged Ethiopia like so many African nations, but we still see it. I smiled at her, making a point of greeting her with my hands as well, the skin of my palm on the skin of her shoulder. I wanted her to know, from this moment, the first time we were meeting, that she was welcome here. As I did so, I remembered with chagrin a much younger version of myself, afraid to share a mattress with Engeda, a student like me and also HIV positive, for fear that the bedbugs or mosquitoes would carry it to me. I know better, now.

With eyes downcast and a voice so gentle I had to move my chair closer to catch her words, Tsega introduced herself and gave her story. She had contracted HIV after her stay in a hospital many weeks' travel away, while receiving treatment for injuries sustained after a road accident had severed the arteries running the length of her thigh. She didn't know which needle it was that had carried the virus into her body, but wondered if it was the blood transfusion. I stifled a gasp as she lifted her dress to show me the extensive scarring. It was incredible she had survived. When her positive status became known in the community, she had no choice but to flee, helped by her mother, who was heartbroken at her daughter's leaving but determined to protect her from further harm. Some months later she had made her way to Cheha Woreda, found work making *injera*, secured a small room to rent and found the son of the landlord looking at her shyly, as she looked back, just as shyly. Some months after that, she was sitting having her hair braided, her hands tracing the beautiful designs embroidered in shades of green on the gauzy white *tibab* she was wearing to marry him. Sitting next to her was her beloved mother, tears in her eyes and hope in her heart. Tsega's whole demeanour changed as she spoke of her husband, a *bajaj* driver in the town, her face melting and the bashfulness fading. When I asked for his name, it clicked into place.

'Tsega, I was at your wedding! I know why I recognise you. My brother, he has a *bajaj* also. We went together.'

She smiled mischievously at me. It suited her. 'I know, Sister Atsede. Tamru told my husband to bring me here.'

'Well, I'd never tell him, but he's a clever man that Tamru. I'm happy you're here. And I'm happy we can look after you with this baby. I want you to know, you don't need to be frightened for your baby. We have medicine that, if you make sure you give it properly, will stop the HIV being passed on. Like the medicine you are taking that is stopping it from being passed to your husband. You're taking medicine, aren't you?' She nodded. 'Good. In a few months, we will buy your baby's medicine together, then keep it here at the Clinic, so you know it's safe. We can also help you, Tsega, with getting to the hospital for the tests you'll need, and to the pharmacy for the medicine you take.'

Being able to say things like this, things that seem so simple but that will so tangibly change Tsega's life, taking away any concern over whether she can afford the travel to the hospital, or the costs associated with the testing, still moves me almost to tears each time. It wasn't so long ago that my father struggled to buy his own medication, to stabilise his blood pressure and control his asthma. I saw, and lived with, the toll the worrying took. While the actual treatment for HIV is provided by the Ministry of Health, mostly free of charge, there are side-effects that need different medications, which are not covered. It is because of an NGO called Ethiopiaid, Indie has told me, that it is possible for me to make these judgements, to offer help to those who need it. The same NGO meant we could travel with Selamawit and her Liyu to Addis

Ababa to meet with the surgeons from America. If I am ever awake at night, lying curled around Mesmora as he sleeps beside me, with the blissful sleep of children worn out from a day's play, I think of this organisation, and the filaments of web that connect the existence of the people working there with the people living here, the net being woven through time and space to link us through these experiences. And now Tsega has her own thread twined in, her own story to add to the anthology.

Tsega laughed in disbelief, unsure whether to trust she had heard me correctly. The tears that I felt in my own eyes were suddenly in hers, and she reached out to take my hand, squeezing it, unable to find the words.

'Sister Atsede, thank you. You don't know what this mea-', her voice broke.

Smiling in gentle understanding, I squeezed back. 'I do, Tsega. I know what this means. We'll look after you. And, when the time comes, your baby too.'

Tsega stood and moved away for a moment, gathering herself. When she turned back, her eyes were bright, and her voice was strong again. The next half an hour passed with much laughter. Without the shadows of fear for her baby or the constant, underlying concerns about managing her own disease casting their shade, her natural vitality, and the enthusiasm for the life she had built in Gubrye, shone through. Her lively energy was infectious, and I felt myself still smiling as I waved Tsega farewell.

Now finished for the evening, I wondered if Indie and I would get home before the rains started. The thunder rumbling ominously in the distance did nothing to reassure me that we would, and I could hear Desu chopping more and more wood, expecting a cold night. As the first drops started to fall, with the distinctive *plink* of rain falling on the corrugated metal roofs, I thought I heard voices talking at the gate. Finishing filing away the patient records, and closing the wooden shutters of the Maternal Health Room against the steadily increasing rain, the voices moved to the room next door, the Birth Room. I wondered if it was just Desu and Indie taking shelter, but as I pulled the door behind me and tried to see through the downpour, I could just make out Desu sitting by the now brightly burning fire. He saw me looking and gestured pointedly at the Birth Room, mouthing something not entirely clear through the deluge.

Keeping as close to the white-washed walls, and as far from the splashing of the cascading water as possible, I edged around the bench and slipped into the Birth Room. The familiar face of Mahaza turned in my direction, a thick blanket pulled over her shoulders. Indie was next to her, shaking the water from her hair.

'The storm is definitely here. Mahaza! What a night.' Even as I said it, the rain intensified, hammering down. I thought briefly of the boys and Yordannos, glad the storm had broken and knowing they'd sleep well with the sounds of it. Mahaza laughed, but it soon faded to a groan as her contractions came. I knew Mahaza well enough to tease her about yet another birth, remembering her fifth, a girl, who I had reached out to catch just last year, her fourth, the year before, her third, her second, and her first, stretching back over my years as a midwife. She was as thin now as she had been then, her abdomen huge by comparison. But it was deceptive, I knew, with her babies all coming along smaller than expected. So far, at least, I thought ruefully.

It was only a handful of days ago that I had seen Mahaza for her final antenatal appointment. Her baby, I recalled now, had been breech. Feeling for the baby's head, back, and legs now, this hadn't changed. The news was greeted with a hopeful smile from Indie, who, I knew, would enjoy the chance to be the leading midwife for Mahaza. In her country, she had told me often, breech is considered very risky, and often becomes a caesarean. I still didn't really believe her, only ever having thought of breech as a different variation, but not so different from those babies born with a hand by their head, or with their faces to the sky. It was true, I conceded as we talked about it, that sometimes breech births needed help, particularly if it was the first baby, but the same is the case for a whole range of different moments in birth, and it didn't necessarily make it an emergency. Mahaza would be happy to for Indie to lead; I knew they had a good rapport.

As the night deepened, Mahaza's body and baby continued their journey through the labour, each contraction softening her cervix, bringing the baby ever further down. As I walked at her side, taking over from Indie who was now sitting with her legs curled up in the chair, idly flicking through a textbook while crocheting cord ties between her fingers, I used the lulls in contractions to ask Mahaza about her husband.

'He is at the *luxor* in Emdibir. There was *minim*, nothing, today, so I told him to go!' She shook her head, then shrugged. 'But Tishi is looking after the children at home, and it means I don't have to worry about getting him breakfast tomorrow, so it isn't all bad.'

I laughed. Mahaza's husband had been there for the last baby, keeping vigil on the bench outside, drinking *kawa* with the guard Seyfu. Both he, and then Mahaza when Indie confessed what she had done, had recoiled in horror when Indie asked whether he would like to come in for the birth. Some couples were open to the idea, but Mahaza and her husband were not among them. The whine of a mosquito passed by, and I reached out to swat it away before catching Indie's eyes and pointing to the incense. Nodding in understanding, the room was soon filled with fragrant smoke of *itane*.

As the next few contractions passed, Mahaza's movements, and the way she held herself, changed. It was time. Indie took her place sitting behind Mahaza, who had dropped down into a deep squat and was now bearing down. Smiling with encouragement at Mahaza, I sat in front of her and spoke as she continued to push. The contraction passed, and came again. Another boy then, I thought, grinning as the evidence of the baby's sex was the first part of his body to emerge. As more of his body came down, I saw Indie's hands go out, then wait, hovering just below the baby. She looked at me for confirmation of her intention to just allow the baby to come, rather than reaching up to turn his body, and inside Mahaza, to release his arms. I agreed. Mahaza needed no help here.

Mahaza's face became a grimace once more as the palms of her hands flattened onto the floor, bracing as she pushed. The relief that swept across her face with that final effort told me all I needed to know. Her son was born. Indie passed the baby, covered in creamy white vernix, through to Mahaza, who at last relaxed from the position she had held through the intensity of birth.

'Well, that wasn't so bad after all,' Mahaza said, winking at me as she helped her baby latch for the first time. She glanced down, wincing slightly as he started to suck, the arm supporting his body holding him close. Without meaning to, my hands went to my own breasts, remembering the sting of the first few days of a baby suckling. Indie grinned as she caught my movement, nodding in agreement. We both looked back to Mahaza, her eyes closed now, resting. More than half an hour passed before she winced again, more noticeably this time, and opened her eyes.

'Feels like a contraction, again?' Mahaza nodded, pursing her lips. 'That could well be the placenta coming away, Mahaza. Stay where you are, leaning back is just fine, and let me have a quick look.'

Minutes later, I closed the lid on the small red bucket that held Mahaza's placenta, and would keep it safe until it was buried in the morning. At the hospitals, the placentas were burnt now, but I could never quite come to terms with that. This miraculous organ, just as complex as any other in our bodies and yet with such a brief timeline, whose entire purpose is to keep the baby alive, reduced to ash? It feels disrespectful somehow, especially when I remember the reverence with which my sister Aklila had treated her own. After her fourth daughter was born at home, when I was still barefoot and not in school, she had dug the hole for the placenta herself, burying it deep within the earth in the corner of our *sahrbet* hut. For years to come, nothing could persuade me to venture there, and the thought of one day accidentally walking over it left me cold with fear. While my dread wasn't shared by my family, the feeling that the placenta was too sacred to desecrate was held by us all. It felt right, now, knowing that the placentas of the Clinic babies were buried, nurturing the earth and giving life to beautiful flowers and spreading trees.

Mahaza's son, content with a belly full of rich yellow colostrum, was sleeping peacefully, his eyelids fluttering occasionally. Gingerly, she folded the hem of her dress in on itself, trying to keep the fluids of the birth, cooled by the night, away from her. I noticed, and called to Desu for another bucket, bigger and blue to differentiate it as containing only water rather than anything else, to be taken to the shower room. As had become habit, the moment a woman came through the gates in labour, Desu would rinse out the huge dented, blackened pot and fill it with clean water, then set it to heat on the flames. A jug of fire-warmed water poured over aching muscles was always welcome after the efforts of birth, but especially on a night like this. Minutes later, clean and dry, having washed in the warm water and donned warm clothes, Mahaza came back into the room with a grateful smile, looking tired but contented. I had finished the checks on her baby and he was sleeping again, having only stirred momentarily when I slipped a gloved finger into his mouth to check for hidden clefts. Leading them to the bed, and ensuring there were enough blankets and a thermos of sweet spicy *chai* within arm's reach, I found Indie moving mats and more blankets around, creating a little nest that would be our bed for the night. Tucked in among the coarse wool, with the *blitchlitch* lights overhead and a sheet pulled over us first to stop it being too itchy, it was warm and peaceful, despite the storm that continued to rage on the other side of the whitewashed mud walls.

The sudden touch of cold caught me by surprise, and I opened my eyes to see that Indie had turned towards me. She had a thoughtful expression on her face, and, like me, didn't look ready to sleep yet. Despite the darkness and lateness, the hours after a birth like Mahaza's always leave me pensive, thinking about this amazing life. It was our relationships with the seasons and the storms, my father used to tell me, with the stars and the land, which were the deciding factors for life itself. As a young girl, I didn't understand fully what he meant, until after he gave me the *frey*, the seed, of an avocado picked from the towering tree in our *gwaro*, and asked me to help it grow. I remember watching anxiously through the hot, rainless months of *berga*, when its leaves browned and curled until I decided to run to the river each morning and bring it water. Just as challenging were the endless soakings it survived through *keremt*, the rains, when I tried to dig holes all around, so the water would run into them instead of sitting at the base of my tree. At the end of that year, I understood what he had been trying to teach me. While my avocado was one of many, and if it failed to produce fruit it would be my pride rather than my hunger that was challenged, I realised how reliant we were on navigating the challenges and offerings of nature in order to survive. It wasn't just growing the avocados and mangoes, or *gomen* or tomatoes, but *enset* too. The waving leaves of the trees could be seen across my village, planted in every *gwaro*, the backbone of Gurage village life. We ate baked *wussa*, made of the leaf sheaths, scraped and left to ferment in pits in the ground, and gummy *gumfo* made from *atameter*, used the fibres to weave mats and string, served our foods in the *ketel*, the leaves, cut into circles and curled into cones. During the harvest, the *gwaro* were alive with the chatter and signing of the women, gathered together to sit on mats on the floor with a leg raised up to rest on the trunk as the scrapers were moved up and down the leaves in tireless movement. While the *enset* were resilient, able to handle the deluge and the drought, many food plants are not as tough, and learning to keep them alive was key to keeping us alive. I hadn't thought of my avocado tree in years, but wondered now how it was handling tonight's storm. My mother, and perhaps my grandmother, must have been awake decades ago wondering the same about their trees. Now the tallest avocado in the village, it had weathered many nights like this, but there would have been a time when its existence was far more precarious.

Turning to Indie, I smiled as I saw her start at the lightning cracking overhead. The storm was right above us now. We spoke, quietly, as I told her about *borja*, the lightning, and about our grandmothers, and their grandmothers, wondering if, perhaps, they had spent nights like this, lying like Indie and I, at the bedside of a woman and her newly born baby, listening to the rain sheeting down. The moments of silence between our words stretched out as we paused, lost in thought, until, eyes closing, I felt the tiredness wash over me and, at last, I slept.

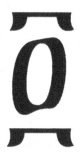

4

Etashy

Indie

The grief of losing a mother must be almost universally dreaded, and even for those of us lucky enough to not have been there, the inconsolable pain all too easy to imagine. Even though Etashy had been very unwell, and her death was a relief from terrible suffering, the tears wept over her shrouded body were real. One day Atsede and I, and our children, will be in Selam's place, burying the beloved women who have been so pivotal in forming and moulding us into the people we become.

As Selam and her sisters stumbled around the room, muttering prayers, their hands clasped at the heart or arms wrapped around themselves as if to keep the crushing sadness from tearing them apart, the village was there, sitting on brightly woven mats around the room, keeping a quiet but constant vigil. No one told them to stop weeping, to control their emotions, that it would be okay. We just sat, lending our presence as they let their grief out. It's an odd thing here, grief: both intensely lonely and entirely shared. The wailing mourning, the *luxor*, started at dawn and will continue through the day, gaining in intensity every time a new group of people arrives and adds their voices, with lulls in between. The sound of sadness reaches out across the *enset* gardens, through the eucalyptus, over the thatched roofs of the *sahrbet* huts ringing the village. Everyone knows death has been there. Seeing the women come, bringing black clay pots used here since time immemorial full of dark, rich *kawa* for the mourners, with white woven scarves wrapped over their heads, the emotional intensity of the *luxor* is inescapable. The elders come together, women with their hands in the air, waving them back and forth to the rhythm of their ululating, men clasping thick carved *dula* sticks with hats pulled low over their eyes. The youngsters too, the girls and boys who grew up playing in Etashy's garden and teasing her cows with long stalks of maize, with black gauzy scarves wrapped around their hair. From all directions, the mourners come.

As well as being our beloved friend, Selam belongs to the same tribe, the same *gowza*, as Atsede, so they are considered family. As kith and kin, we take our places inside the room where Etashy lies, behind a white sheet strung up. It is embroidered with the Gurage cross in rich, earthy tones. I remember Selam making it, letting me place a few stitches, laughing at my attempts. I look for her. In a yellow flowing dress, wooden bangles at her wrists and matching wooden earrings defining her face, her hair braided only yesterday, she is beautiful. The rivulets of tears coursing over her cheeks don't detract from it. She is standing now, silent, bereft, leaning against the wall next to her sisters, Lakech, sitting and rocking back and forth holding their mother's hand, and Amarech, prostrate over their mother's legs, and Addis, caressing the corner of the shroud closest to their mother's head. I catch her attention briefly, and murmur nothing in particular, but knowing she sees my sympathy for her loss. All around the room are eyes with faraway looks, and shoulders shaking gently with sobs. We are all thinking of our own mothers. Although feeling so sad aches, how lucky we are to love someone to the extent that just the thought of their absence can cause it.

Etashy had died in the early hours, so today would also be her burial. As an Ethiopian Orthodox Christian, this would take place in the church in the town nearby. With no roads between the villages and the towns, Etashy's body would go by pick-up, accompanied by her children, holding on to her and to each other. One last journey together. The mourning village processes as one, out of her hut, along the well-trodden paths through the forest, around the gully, across the river, and up the slope to church, which sits high up overlooking the marketplace, teeming with people and livestock. Atsede, her older sisters and I walk together, keeping our *netela* out of the red dust and away from the snags of burrs. It's a beautiful day, the sun shining but an unusual breeze keeping it from being too warm. It's some way to the town, so we have time to talk. I ask about Etashy's early life, which Aklila, the eldest of Atsede's siblings, remembers. 'She was full of laughter, and happiness, always encouraging us to see the beauty in little things, spiders' webs hung with dew, or the feather of a bird. If we'd been naughty, and were afraid of going home, it was Etashy who we went to, begging her to help.' I loved hearing these memories, and could so easily picture Etashy like this rather than as I knew her, already elderly but with a sparkle to her eye, frail but never weak.

With the deterioration of her body through the years, Etashy had been bed-bound for some time, cared for with doting attention by her youngest daughter, Amarech. Rarely sick until her last days, from her bed in the hut, propped up on pillows and covered in the embroidered sheet that now shrouded her coffin, Etashy had nevertheless maintained a presence in the community. At no time was this more apparent than during Meskel, the celebration among the Christians that commemorates the finding of the Cross. For the week-long holiday, when nothing but raw meat, either diced finely and mixed with a spiced, clarified butter as *kutfo* or simply cut off the bone and taken as chunks of *kort*, is eaten, family from all corners of the country return to their homes in the villages. Half way through the week, the *chengya,* the humps, of the zebu cows slaughtered by each household are collected together and brought to Etashy as an offering of solidarity and respect. And then, with the meat prepared by all the village women in Etashy's kitchen, everyone congregates at her bedside with the broad, dark green leaves of the ubiquitous *enset* tree shaped into a cone to receive a share of the delicacy. Over the years, the tradition grew and grew, with each family contributing one thing or another; clay pots of butter churned from the milk of the cows that wander the paths between houses, gourds of home-brewed alcohol, huge rounds of bread baked over the fires perpetually burning in any village kitchen, ready at a moment to roast *kawa* or heat food for visitors. At night, the music starts as the big bonfire burns lower, with singing and dancing into the early hours. It is saddening to think that now Etashy has gone, there is no need to continue this part of the Meskel celebrations so unique to her village. I ask Atsede about it, not sure I want to hear the answer. But no one is quite sure.

The noises of the market: lowing cattle, the bang of metal as machetes are re-shaped and sharpened, and an occasional hollering voice rising above the general rumble of conversation, are coming louder through the trees. We are nearly there. Stopping to break off a few of the small, lower branches of the feathery trees to beat off the inevitable dust that has accumulated around our long dresses and trailing scarves, we straighten our clothes and take deep breaths, readying ourselves for Etashy to be laid in her final resting place. It is the time of *tsomme*, a two-month period of no animal products in the lead up to *Fasika*, Easter, and so the funeral service won't start until late afternoon. We take our places with the women, sitting in small groups on logs and boulders, backs leaning against the trunks of pine trees. It's quiet, peaceful, just the whispering of wind in the canopy of leaves above us and the murmuring of voices. Selam and her family have accompanied the coffin inside, where the priests are chanting and praying in the heavily perfumed air. Until the service is finished, we stay in the cool, dappled shade of the trees, watching the mourners come and go, nodding greetings at those we know, or think we know. And then, to the *macabre boter*, the burial grounds, where the male members of Etashy's *gowza* have been digging the grave. A keening wail rents the air as Amarech leads the procession out of the church. The respite from their grief that came with dedicated prayers and the familiar rhythm of the rituals of the church has broken. The walk through the forest to the graveyard marks the last few moments Etashy's family will have together with her. We fall into place behind Selam, scarves once again over our hair and eyes downcast. And then suddenly it is over, Etashy has been returned to the earth, the red soil heaped over the coffin, and a simple wooden cross marks the place where her head is, aligned to the axis of the church.

Red plastic plates heaped with *injera* and *misr wot*, a thick, spicy dhal-like sauce made with lentils and fresh, sweet tomatoes from the market, are passed around. Women circulate with jerrycans full of cold, clear water, drunk from metal cups they carry in baskets. A last meal to share with Etashy. And then, back along the well-trodden paths through the forest to the village. The nature of the grief in the air and the eyes of Etashy's children has lessened somewhat, as if committing her soul to Heaven and her body to the ground has made it easier to bear. No longer overwrought despair, the tones of the crying have settled into the sounds of missing Etashy, as they always will.

The village will keep vigil now, over the coming days, so Etashy's family will not be alone with their sadness. Atsede and I join them when we can, over the lunchtime period with its lull in patients, in the evenings. Endless cups of strong, bitter *kawa*, plucked from the plants grown across the village gardens, are passed around, along with handfuls of roasted barley and chickpeas. The constant presence of humanity is a background reassurance of life in the face of death, Atsede was explaining as we leaned against the gnarled old tree in Etashy's garden, idly watching a young calf grazing. In our laps we had wide, shallow, woven baskets full of hard, round, dried chickpeas. We were separating them from the grains of different kinds that were inevitably mixed in at the mills. Atsede periodically tipped the sorted chickpeas into her winnowing tray, and tossed them high into the air, letting the breeze carry away the lighter chaff and husks. It was a skill I was still learning, and could only manage with great concentration. Atsede, meanwhile, had continued discussing the merits of the *luxor* without dropping a single pea. The *chah chah* sound the winnowing makes is as distinctive as that of the *thunk* of roasted *kawa* in the process of being pounded, and hearing both is sure indication that a household has guests. Atsede paused, and from the faraway tone of her voice as it faded out, I knew she was remembering her father's death. His widely acknowledged favourite, Atsede had been deeply affected by his passing only a few years ago. As with Selam's grief over the loss of her mother, I am deeply grateful not to have experienced Atsede's grief over the loss of her father. It must be so difficult to suddenly exist in a world where your mother and father do not.

Death is not hidden here. The children are not shielded from the sadness, nor excused from paying their respects where it has visited. As new voices joined the keening, I looked to the wooden door, hanging off just one hinge after a truant zebu kicked it in an attempt to enter the house in search of food. Already dressed in black, and mourning deeply the loss of her own father just a handful of days previously, came the slim figure of Dirshe, the young daughter of Alem, the Clinic's housekeeper and a much-adored friend. Unlike Etashy, whose body had given in to the ravages of illness, it was the mind of Dirshe's father that could not recover. For months we had agonised over how to help Habtu, lamenting the lack of access to mental health services and our own helplessness. An accident some years previously had left him with a slipped disc, unable to work, and only able to move around with great pain. For a man previously full of vitality and an almost restless energy, the loss of his freedom had come at a price. Even over the four years that I had known him he had changed, withdrawn into himself, faded somehow. His mind was still sharp, but overshadowed by something difficult to define. It was almost impossible to imagine him as Atsede and Alem talked of him, full of enthusiastic gesticulations and grand plans, particularly for Dirshe, whom he would tell, time and again, about the huge bull he would buy on the day she decided to marry. Dirshe had laughed delightedly in response, I was told, and chided him for not instead celebrating her graduation from school or university. The warmth between them had always been evident, and the weeks of his decline had, in many ways, been the most difficult for her. Not quite still a child, and able to escape into the worlds of play and make-believe, but not yet a woman, with the responsibilities of hosting guests to provide distraction, Dirshe was left in between, with the full force of her grief. I watched her now, moving between the mourners already leaving the hut, her hand in that of her friend, Reddit, and her eyes holding a sadness too great for a child of her age.

I glanced at Atsede, resting back against the knoll of the tree, a small cup of *kawa* in one hand, and saw her eyes were also following Dirshe. She had felt our failure as much as I did, but also carried a deeper guilt over the frustration she had felt towards Habtu for not being able to help himself. Having sat beside her weeping father as he lay dying in a hospital bed from a combination of diseases his body could no longer keep at bay, Atsede just couldn't comprehend how Habtu had chosen to leave his children, his family, his life. But his suicide wasn't a choice made by a balanced and rational father and husband. It was the desperate last measure of a tormented man trapped in his own mind, unable to see any other way out of the suffering. In the weeks leading up to his death, Atsede, Aster and I had spent hours sitting on the low bamboo chairs lining the waiting area of our Clinic, the conversations going back and forth over what we could do. And it was always with apprehension that we greeted Alem as she arrived in the morning, dreading the news of how the family had coped through the night.

Over what would be, although we didn't know it then, the last few weeks of his life, Habtu had needed someone with him day and night. In the rare moments he was alone, while his keeper ran to the latrine pits in the cool dark of dawn, or drifted to sleep in the heat of the sun, Habtu had made increasingly desperate attempts to take his own life. It was with a piercing guilt that we heard of his daughter cutting him from the tree in the garden, or his son binding his wrists with lengths of *enset* leaf. It soon became difficult enough to meet each other's eyes, and all but impossible to meet Alem's. As we walked home at the end of the day, our children dozing on our backs, the same thoughts were woven through tired, dispirited conversations. We were clinicians, nurses and midwives, trained and qualified to be there for those in need of care. And more than that, we ran a medical centre and spent our days immersed in providing treatment. Yet now we were in a position where we were utterly lost, helpless and unable to do anything to bring Habtu back from the edge of the precipice.

The most difficult day, perhaps even more so than the day he drowned, was the day we crouched around Habtu, huddled under a blanket, cross-legged and blank-eyed, and tried to explain, to justify why his hands were now bound at the wrist. In the quietest, darkest moments of night, while we sat, backs leaning against the cool white walls of the Clinic's veranda as women traced paths over the mosaic of tiles bathed in moonlight, groaning through each contraction, Atsede and I had whispered to each other, wondering if, at that moment you tie on shackles, there is actually a rush of feeling of invincible power. To be in a position of complete control over another human being, to decide their moves – we pondered whether there were vestiges of enough primal wildness in us to make that satisfying. And yet, when the moment came, we realised just how wrong we had been. It was with nothing but a deep and desolate sadness, lost for words and holding back tears, that we stood by as Habtu's wrists were tied. The decision to deprive another human being of liberty, the most basic and fundamental right, regardless of how good and just the intentions, carries an inexplicable weight. It was felt in the deepest part of our souls, and there was just enough room left in our hearts to feel anger alongside the sadness, anger that without the means to medically guard Habtu from himself, we had no choice but to do it physically. I reached out to colleagues around the world, asking for guidance, for help, for an answer as to how we could save Habtu. The response was overwhelming in its kindness and understanding, with no judgement for the steps we'd taken, but great sympathy. Dr Moore, a British consultant psychologist, lent the weight of her decades of experience in crisis situations, and for a time a subdued hope pervaded the air.

But we had no medication, we had no cognitive behaviour therapy or counselling. We had no options, no way to bring him out of the darkness. And when it all became too much for Alem, no longer able to bear the strain on the faces of her children, Habtu was carried to the church, where he would spend the next fortnight going through ritual purifications, exorcisms, and spiritual cleansings. There were brief moments of lucidity, but over time these proved not to be steps along the path to recovery, but instead the calm before the storm. Each time he fell, it was harder and harder to hold him up. Alem lost weight, her clothes hanging from her once robust frame, and her mind was never away from Habtu, even when she was at work. We gave her as much time off as she asked for, but as the days slipped into weeks she needed the respite of mornings at the Clinic, the tranquillity of the swaying trees full of butterflies, of swishing a mop over the white-tiled floors, and the distraction of bursts of laughter from us all, watching as my son learnt how to crawl and Atsede's son learnt how to help him. But these were fleeting moments of relief, and each afternoon she would return to the dilapidated hut in the grounds of the Orthodox church. Until one day, when she returned and he wasn't there. He had slipped through the safety net we had so diligently been holding taut, and, just like that, it was all over.

The news of his death, in the calm waters of the river that meanders through the marketplace before traversing the length of the mountain range, came that afternoon. Atsede was sitting with a woman who had come wondering if the tight feelings across her bump were the start of labour, while I had ushered our sons, crawling and toddling, into the shade of the waiting area, distracting them with a torch, flicking it on and off and casting dancing light across the corrugated iron roofing. Diego, my son's father, had arrived earlier in the week and was soaking up the sunlit hours spent laughing with his son. It had been a gentle, peaceful afternoon, as we gathered around the clay *jebena* pot between patients, feeding the babies handfuls of roasted barley and relaying to Diego tales of the boys' antics over the last few months. As ever, it takes only a moment for it all to change. It was Aster who took the phone call from Mekdes, Atsede's sister. I heard her call out from the Emergency Room, where she had been folding gauze, preparing it for the autoclave, balanced precariously over the rocks that ringed the fireplace, and looked at Diego, raising an eyebrow. Handing the baby, whose eyes had become heavy with sleep after nursing, over, I stretched and stood up. As I walked up the veranda, I could hear more of the conversation, and felt my heartbeat quicken along with my steps. On the way past, I pushed open the wooden door to the Maternal and Child Health Room, apologising for interrupting but asking Atsede to come with me for a moment to the Emergency Room. Addis, the young woman who lived next door to Atsede and I, and was now expecting her second child, a little over two years after I was there to catch her first daughter, was comfortable, sitting on the birth ball that rolled inexplicably around the Clinic with a mind of its own, turning up in the most unexpected places. She smiled in agreement as she heard my request, and waved a hand dismissing Atsede's apologies. As I turned, I felt Atsede catch my hand.

'Indie, what's going on, there isn't a patient in the Emergency Room?'

Just as I opened my mouth to answer, Aster stepped out in front of us. Her eyes were wide and she was staring at the phone still held aloft. There was a moment, just a moment, before she confirmed what we both suspected. In it, I looked around at the little world we'd created in the Clinic, at the flowering trees, the diffuse sunshine, the butterflies, our sons, and their fathers, preparing to take on the reality of Alem's loss, of our loss. The rest of the afternoon was fractured, some minutes disappearing, some lasting forever. Diego would stay with the boys at home as, for the first time since the Clinic had been opened, we locked the gates while the sun was still up. Back at the house, we found the gauzy, white *nutella* shawls, worn to church, to weddings, to funerals, and made our way, mostly in silent disbelief, to the road. On the way, we stopped to buy handfuls of *kawa* beans to take, knowing that already, within minutes of the news of Habtu's death, their hut would be full of mourners, all of whom would need the rich, fortifying warmth to face the grief of the new widow and her children. While Aster and I were deeply saddened, as I watched Atsede climb into the *bajaj* ahead of me, I saw her eyes were haunted with guilt as well as sadness. Her stoicism through the difficulties of her life had left Atsede with a belief in the power we all have to accept our circumstances and make the most of them. Over the last few weeks, Atsede had become increasingly frustrated with Habtu's behaviour, unable to see this wasn't the man she had grown up knowing, who had brought her small gifts as a child, and worked alongside her at the hospital. She saw the pain in Alem, and in their daughter and sons, and blamed him. I knew her reaction was caught up not only in the loss of her own father, but also in the deaths of the women and babies under her care. The memories of them stayed with her, and her anger at Habtu was as much at herself for not being able to save him, save any of them, as it was at his inability to endure the difficult times in the hope of better times to come.

In the months to come, it was her work at the Clinic, Alem said, that sustained her. The antics of Mesmora and Raphael, as they discovered how to prize the tops off jerrycans and fill them with stones, causing Aster to chase them up and down the veranda, pretending to threaten them with a sugarcane. The old women who came with no money, but baskets of eggs or jars of honey in return for treatment, and the young women who came with their baby in their belly and left with their baby in their arms. A gift also came in the form of Selam's youngest child, her three-year-old daughter Reddit, who had returned from Addis Ababa much improved after a stressful few months of uncertainty. She often joined our boys at the Clinic as Selam stayed with her mourning family in the village overseeing the *luxor*, and loved nothing more than sitting as close as she could to Alem, passing her petals from flowers or little *jebena* she'd shaped from mud. In the first weeks of Reddit's undiagnosed illness, we'd cared for her at the Clinic, drawing bloods and sending them to the hospital for investigations, until it became apparent that whatever was wrong stretched far beyond our abilities to look after her.

'You were right', Selam had said, turning to me. Just a week before her mother's death, which would take her away from the town for days on end, we were sitting on her veranda, on carved wooden *burchama* stools, trying to entice the last few wisps of evening breeze to cool our sun-baked babies, watching the chickens scratch at the dirt for insects, 'it's idiopathic thrombocytopenic purpura, ITP'. Thank God, I thought to myself, utterly relieved that little Reddit hadn't been diagnosed with the other, far more sinister, disease of the blood that her symptoms pointed to.

A gentle soul, Selam may not be quite as outspoken as Atsede and I, but her quick mind and affectionate sense of humour often left us in peals of laughter, wiping tears from cheeks and trying to catch our breath. There hadn't been much laughter recently, though. Even before the death of her mother, the Sunday visits that had become ritual after Atsede and I left our posts at the hospital were punctuated by the same worried conversation going back and forth. Reddit's haemoglobin was low, leaving her listless and pale, and her platelets, the cells in the body responsible for helping the blood to clot, were less than 10% of what they should be. What was going on inside her was hidden, out of sight, like a malevolent shadow just visible out of the corner of our eyes, but with all too evident effects.

It had started slowly. A fortnight or so of bruises appearing all over her little body, the result of the innocuous bumps that come with learning to crawl and walk. A rash-like mark, petechaie, forming under the waistband of a pair of leggings or the cuff of a wrist. And, one difficult night, a nosebleed that had us rushing to her house in the dark, afraid of the hyenas but even more afraid of Selam's frantic phone call that it wouldn't stop.

The next morning, before the sun had even fully risen, Selam and her daughter had started the journey to Addis Ababa. The hospital here didn't have the necessary levels of knowledge, equipment, or experience to work out what was going on. As we sat with Selam until the cool dawn, soaking towels in cold water and passing her new ones, murmuring reassurances we didn't fully believe, with Reddit continuing to drip blood, I had sent a ream of emails back to the UK, fervently grateful that internet, although entirely unreliable, was at that moment functional. The benefit of a friendship with an emergency doctor working at Addenbrookes Hospital in Cambridge, whom I had known since before he had even started medical school, was the network of other specialist doctors that came with him. I heard from several and the overwhelming response was to get her to a hospital. ITP, among others, was suggested, and seemed the favoured diagnosis, but regardless of what it was, bleeding was dangerous. She needed to be seen.

Many days later, by which time Selam was wrung out and Reddit fed up of the prick of needles, we had an answer. During her stay at the Black Lion Hospital, a huge, sprawling complex in the capital, Reddit had not only had countless rafts of blood tests, but also bone marrow aspirations, lumbar punctures, and various imaging studies. In the midst of all that came unit after unit of whole blood and platelets to try and bring her own levels to something resembling normal. So much time for a child who previously just wanted to move and play and dance and laugh to be still. Selam's voice shook with the effort of keeping tears in check as she described Reddit's fragile cries as yet another gloved and masked nurse came with needles and syringes. My heart clenched in sympathy as I cuddled my son close, unable to imagine how difficult it must be to see your child spending days in a paediatric ward. It was hard enough knowing Selam and Reddit were there.

Our main concern now, with her relentlessly low platelet levels despite the transfusions, is the risk of intracranial haemorrhage. As the little sister of a rambunctious four-year-old, being knocked over occasionally is part of life. But with Reddit's spleen playing havoc, destroying her healthy platelets as well as the older ones, if she were to fall the wrong way and hit her head, the consequences could be devastating. This type of thrombocytopenia has no cure, and although it's often self-limiting, until she has reliably stable test results, we won't breathe easy.

Though her tiny body was still struggling, her time under the watchful eye of the doctors in Addis Ababa had wrought a significant change on sleepy Reddit. In part thanks to her slowly recovering haemoglobin levels, but also a reflection of her natural vitality as a young child hardwired to survive, Reddit was once again full of bubbling energy. Her appetite was back, as was her cheeky attitude. Selam seemed calmer too, or perhaps just with a stronger sense of resolve. The air was pervaded by a sense of subdued hope and cautious optimism. And every test that came back showing stable or marginally improved numbers contributed towards that feeling.

After taking several weeks of leave to be with Reddit, Selam was once again back on the delivery ward. We had no idea then that she would soon be walking out of the doors to the hospital for another two weeks.

Having talked through every minute detail of her daughter's treatment, and reassured ourselves that Reddit was getting the best care possible, our conversation turned, as it often did, to midwifery. We smiled over our more entertaining shifts together, full of laughter and love and friendship and healthy new lives, and commiserated over the more difficult ones, the supplies we ran out of and the patients we couldn't save. As our children, tired of balancing stones on bricks, started to get restless in a way that can only be resolved with sleep, we slung them on to our backs and went for a twilight walk, unwilling to call it a night.

It was the season for fireflies, and Selam laughed delightedly into the cool evening air as I stood, captivated by the tiny glowing lights. We talked about Habtu, about how exhausting it was for Alem and her children, about the helplessness we felt about not knowing what to do next. There was little more to say though, and no answers to unearth. We talked instead about the Clinic, about the women Atsede and I had helped birth over the weeks Selam was away, and about the patients coming to the Emergency Room who kept us just as busy. We had had midwives from America visiting not that long ago, I was telling Selam, bringing all sorts of fantastic bits of equipment, not least of which was an ultrasound machine, which we were using happily every day. I regaled her with tales of how Atsede and I had been trying to show women the features of their little babies, hands and noses and feet, only for them to panic and wonder why their baby's skin was such a strange colour, and worry that their babies would be delivered looking like that. For women who have little exposure to ultrasound, it must be very difficult to see a soft, warm, breathing baby in the grey shades of a scan. We carried on though, with all the time in the world to sit with each woman, cooing over their baby's kicking legs and beating hearts. We pointed out the sucking movements as the baby swallows amniotic fluid, and the bones of the spine and rib cage, the fists that clenched around the umbilical cord.

There is a certain reluctance here to become too emotionally involved in a pregnancy, and even in the early days of the baby's life. It is a protective barrier and the result of generations of women who have lost children. Even now, neonatal mortality rates are shockingly high. Two young doctors came to the hospital to collect data on this just a few years ago, and were saddened to find that of every 1,000 babies born, almost 200 will die in their first 28 days. As they wrote up their reports, they stayed in rooms next to mine, so I had the opportunity to talk to them about the reasons behind the statistics, the lack of infrastructure, the poverty, the distance from health facilities, too few midwives and too many women. The staff at the hospital, who live this reality day in and day out, were shocked but not surprised at the high number. Change will come, and already has in many ways, but it's a slow, gradual process relying on many different aspects coming together. Even so, each midwife has a part to play, and each baby guided into the world healthy is a victory worth recognition against this backdrop of heartbreak.

A lull in the conversation as we walked, no doubt brought on by my mind wandering away from whatever Selam had been saying, was interrupted when she spoke up.

'I made Tensu's *ajah*.' I frowned, mid-step, and turned to Selam. 'Tensu's *ajah*? What do you mean?'

'He still isn't talking, you know that. So, I made him *ajah*. To help him talk.'

That provided no clarity, and I was as lost as ever as to what Selam meant. I knew about *ajah*, of course, it was the nutrient-dense, porridge-like drink made from grains and seeds and nuts roasted then pounded, and mixed with hot water and honey, ubiquitous at the bedside of *chyne*, postnatal, mothers, sipped throughout the day for sustenance and to help encourage milk supplies. *Ajah* was wonderful in this context, full of minerals, vitamins, proteins and fibre, as well as providing the sweetness and medicinal properties of honey. But I'd never heard of it helping a young child to talk. Selam could see my confusion, and smiled kindly.

'You didn't know this?' I shook my head, confirming her suspicions. 'Well, if you have a child who isn't talking, then you have to go to the *geya*, the market, and ask for just one grain of each variety from every merchant. You can't buy it; it has to be given to you. And then, when you've collected all of those, you take them home, and make *ajah* from what you have. The child drinks the *ajah*, and learns to talk.'

'Oh,' I knew that Selam, for all her serenity and calmness in the face of challenges, had started to grow a little concerned that Tensu, now almost five, was still not talking, 'And? Is it working?'

'Not yet, but it might.' She sounded a little dejected, but when she spoke next, it was full of happiness. 'But he does say 'Kibe' and 'Ser' all the time now, rather than just sometimes, like before.'

'Ser?'

'Selam.'

'And "Kibe", that must be Kibebe?' Kibebe, Selam's husband, Tensu's father, worked at the maintenance department at the hospital. He had wired the Clinic's electricity in place, and could often be found up a hastily bashed together wooden ladder, pliers dangling from one hand, and a collection of wires and cable around his waist and over his shoulder. A rotund, jolly man, always smiling and yelling out greetings to whoever happens to walking by, he was a fine match for Selam, and an adored playmate to his children. Selam nodded in response.

'That's great, Selam. He'll get there.' I smiled with affection as I remembered his insistent gestures for me to peel his mango earlier, and his shy kiss on my check when I handed it over, 'And anyway, he might not talk, but he communicates just fine. He's a good boy, Selam. The words will come.'

I wonder if she ever looked back on those worries now she was dealing with the loss of Etashy, whether she would think it seemed so insignificant now that she had been so bothered about her healthy, happy, joyful son who simply didn't say as many words as others. In the weeks of Etashy's *luxor,* when we greeted her with soft words and gentle touches in the evening as she came to find Reddit and take her home, she never mentioned Tensu's lack of speech, instead just repeating her gratefulness to have her children with her at night, curled up next to her on their mattress on the floor. No matter what age you are, without parents you are still an orphan, she had said to us.

Time, as with so many things, didn't reduce Selam's sadness, but helped her to find a way to live with it. As it did for Alem. And before we knew it, she came to the Clinic one morning not in the black clothes of a widow that we had grown so accustomed to, but in a yellow top and blue skirt. It was jarring to think that a year had already passed. The mourning period was over. It was time to live in colour again. I noticed, one day, weeks after I became used to seeing the reds and greens of dresses that had been folded away in the wooden trunk for so many months, that she still wears a black *shajsh* bound around her hair. I asked Atsede about it, quietly, one day as we passed blue folders between us, making sure they went back on to the shelves that held them in the correct order.

'She wears colour, because she no longer has to mourn him, but she wears black, because she's still allowed to miss him.' Atsede had said, quietly.

Atsede

Had it really been only yesterday that we had visited Etashy? The room had changed so much since then. Even her ever-present bed had already been moved elsewhere, replaced instead by her coffin. Along with sharing in the sadness of her daughters, my sisters from our *gowza*, our tribe, the Ergah, I carried a weight that few knew of. In the weeks leading up to Etashy's death, as her body slowly gave in to a lifetime of hardships, I had not made the time to take *kawa*, or food, or just a smile. My living had taken me from Etashy's dying. The guilt sat heavy on my shoulders, and as I wept, the tears were of regret as much as grief. The consolation that we were here yesterday, to say farewell one last time, did little to assuage it. She had forgiven me, though, after the wicked smile that so often flashed across her features had accompanied her teasing that I had forgotten all about her. Her charisma was undiminished, despite her declining body. I had smiled in return, hearing the waver in her voice as she spoke, knowing what the almost translucent quality to her skin meant. It wouldn't be long now, I thought, until you can rest. Etashy, and her family, had played a quiet but ever-present role in my life in the village, and I had spent more sunlit afternoons sitting on the same mat on her hard-packed floor that now held the mourners than I could remember.

All I have to do is close my eyes and I'm back in that moment, five years ago. It was Rahel who told me. She had just come on duty, and had heard the keening of my brother and sister, on their knees at the bedside of my father. 'Come, Atsede', she had said, 'wash your hands, and come.'

I wasn't there for his death, because I was at a birth. In that one moment, the past and the future collided. My hands were barely dry from the water that had carried away vernix, the evidence of birth, when they touched the cooling skin of my father, the evidence of death. It was an unnerving feeling, to have stepped out of the room that saw it all begin and into the room that saw it all end. But in the next heartbeat, my grief drove out everything else. It was despair like I hadn't known. I couldn't breathe, I couldn't think. My father was gone. It has been years now, but at every *luxor* it is as if no time at all has passed, and Etashy's was no different. But alongside the sadness, I felt an upswelling of pride in the villages, in the Gurage people. Whenever we were needed, whatever time of day or night, wherever we had to be, we came. In a time and a place where death occurs all too often, we have learnt the lessons from our ancestors: grief is easier to bear if we are together.

I looked around the room, full of the men and women I had grown up with, catching an eye and exchanging sad nods of acknowledgement, before searching for Selam, for Addis, for Lakech. Etashy's daughters were grouped together now, sitting and squatting quietly, accepting the gentle murmuring condolences that came their way. The older women lined one side of the room, sitting shoulder to shoulder on colourful woven mats, hands clasped on their knees drawn up in front of them. Some had their chins resting there, *nutella* scarves enclosing them completely. A breeze came though the perpetually opened wooden doors and windows, but it did little to cool the room, full of bodies and movement, and under the glare of the midday sun. On the chairs against the opposite walls sat the men, their worn *dula* sticks laid neatly at their feet, thick *gabi* thrown over their shoulders, hats pulled low over their eyes. Closest to the door, in the position saved for those who commanded the most respect, sat my father-in-law, Geremew, the village chief. He watched the proceedings solemnly, and I wonder how it felt for him as, more and more often, it was the *luxor* of his contemporaries that he was attending now. His wife, Dawit's mother Bizunesh, had been unwell for some time, an underlying problem with her heart that no medicine seemed to heal. Was he thinking of her? I murmured a greeting in his direction as his eyes, full of sorrow and understanding, met mine. He nodded in acknowledgement, then resumed his solemn stare into his hands, gnarled and knotted, resting on his lap. A memory, from the last time I had seen Etashy while she was well, came to me suddenly. It had been raining all night, and the tracks to the village were muddy and slick. Despite that, the boys had begged us to take them to see Abate Geremew, as he was known to the youngsters, and his new calf, born in the night. On the way back, we had passed Etashy's *sahrbet* and ducked in, the boys laughing and jostling to be placed on the bed next to her, a prize position. With the *kawa* passed around now finished, and the first drops of rain making the distinctive *plink* on the sheet metal roof, we had waved farewell to Etashy and made our way through her *gwaro* to the path that would eventually take us back to the road. Slipping and sliding in the mud, grabbing wildly onto the tough stalks of *qat* that grew alongside the *enset,* avocados, and coffee, it was with little grace that we navigated the steep hill. With the carefree laughter of children, the boys had flung themselves down the slope without a thought, just as happy to end up on their knees or backsides as they were on their feet. I very nearly toppled over altogether, then I heard our names called. Gliding down the path, barefoot and supremely unfazed, as if the mud didn't even exist, was Geremew. He soon overtook us, sparing just a moment to watch, with undisguised amusement, as Indie tried to set me back on my feet without losing her own balance. It was a story that Indie had taken great pleasure in retelling once we were safely back at the Clinic, how elderly Geremew had bounded past us without so much as backward glance. 'It kept happening,' she would lament, reminding us of a time just a few weeks previously, when we had taken a kilo of meat to my mother to celebrate Adwa, the battle that took place in the mountains to the north when the barefoot, spear-wielding warriors of the highlands had beaten off the Italian invaders. After helping to prepare the spicy *kutfo* and sitting to eat together in the bright sunshine, we had started over the grasslands, talking as we meandered, only to find my mother soon passing us on her way to the *geya,* market.

'Do you intend to get home tonight, my daughters?' she had asked, smiling with a teasing affection.

Back in the present, I looked more closely at the small figures of the older women leaning against the wall, wondering if my mother was among them. I couldn't see her, but the group of younger women who had just arrived were moving through the empty space left in the middle, their hands in the air, moving in time to their wails, obscuring the rest of the room. Even if she was not here now, she would have been here earlier, I was sure. The familiar sounds of pleas to God came from the group of women, not for deliverance from the pain of grief, but for peace for Etashy in the afterlife. Most of our village was Catholic, and while the voice of the muezzin singing out from the small mosque serving just two families joined the church bells that tolled on a Sunday, the sounds of the *luxor* were Christian. Etashy, though, was Orthodox, and it was because of this that through the door now appeared a man dressed in a crisp white tunic that fell to his knees, white trousers visible beneath, with a length of white cloth bound around his head as a turban. In one hand he held a tarnished, beaten silver cross, in the other a worn Bible, written I recognised in the ancient Geez language of the Orthodox Church. Around his neck was a dark leather cord, dangling from which I was certain was a scripture from the Bible, written by hand onto a scrap of paper then folded in on itself time and again until it could be encased in a strip of leather and bound to the necklace, lying directly over his breastbone, the brown-black a stark contrast to the white. Indie had asked, more than once, as we sat side-by-side on a Sunday afternoon, hands immersed in soapy water, scrubbing mud stains from the hems of our own white *tibeb,* why the clothes of the Church were white in a country where there was always either red dust or even redder mud. I laughed at her exasperation, but it stayed in my mind. Watching Abba, the priest glowing in the warm sunshine, walk in, I caught a glimpse of why. It was a way to show our commitment to our faith. *Look,* we say, dressed in white, *look, God, at how important you are to us, look at how much effort we put into these beautiful clothes that shroud our beautiful bodies, bodies You made. Look, at these imperfect souls striving to live a life of meaning despite our shortcomings, despite the poverty, the diseases, the starvation. Look, at our faith and our hope and our fortitude. Look, and bless us, and guide us, and love us.*

Along with the fresh air that came as Abba opened the door to move into the room, so too came the scent of roasting *kawa,* and the sound of the thudding as thick wooden poles were pounded into the waist-high wooden mortar to keep up with the constant stream of mourners. Women flitted between the cooking huts, where rings of stone contained flickering fires, and the orchards, stacked with wood collected in the early hours in anticipation of the coming days, their long dresses trailing behind them and their hair bound in brightly-coloured scarves. Their faces were solemn, but they moved with purpose. The role of ensuring there is enough of the roasted barley and fresh *kawa* in the first days, and dishes of sour, fermented *injera* served with spicy *wot* in the days to come, falls to the young women, unwed and so often still living in the village, the pull of the towns not yet luring them away from their family's homes. With the women taking over the hosting duties, the family can mourn.

In time, towards the end of the day, Etashy would be borne on the back of a pick-up across the *meda,* the grasslands, through the forest, and down the gulley. From there, she would travel along the track that led from the hospital to the road, then along the road to the graveyard of the church, sitting like a sentinel atop the hill overlooking the *geya,* the market. Not in decades had she been so far from the mud walls of the *sahrbet.* I couldn't remember a time when Etashy had walked, but Aklila, my oldest sister, did. I couldn't remember, either, what had robbed her of that faculty. From what I'd heard though, she'd been working in the *gwaro* one day, preparing the *enset* for transplanting, a ritual that happened every year for seven years until it was ready to be processed. That evening she'd fallen ill, slipped into unconsciousness. She wasn't taken to the hospital; trust in medicine was still in its infancy all those years ago, but was cared for at home. My mother had been among the women there. When Etashy awoke, she could simply no longer move anything more than her head. Perhaps it was an overwhelming, fast-moving infection that had eaten away at her spinal column, a doctor had postulated some years later when Dr Rita had taken him to visit her for an unrelated reason, whether fungal or bacterial he couldn't be sure. Or maybe she'd had a stroke. There was no answer, but Etashy simply accepted her new fate. The *sheyhr,* the shaman, had come, as had the *shagwara,* the sorcerer. Neither of them, though, had any more answers. Etashy had huffed at the retreating back of the *shagwara.*

'Idiot man', she had said, 'I never liked him.'

Her daughters had looked at her, aghast, terrified she was calling upon herself all sorts of malevolence. Their hands were a blur as they rushed to cross themselves, muttering prayers under their breath. I had had to suppress a giggle, admiring and adoring her candour in equal measure.

'*Emar!* Mother!' Amarech, her youngest daughter, who had given her whole life to care for Etashy, exclaimed, 'You can't say that.'

Etashy had harrumphed. 'I'll say what I please. Anyway, you didn't see what depraved advice he gave the sweet son of Getachew. "Sacrifice a donkey," that old *shagwara* had said,' Etashy put on an exaggerated voice, low and gravelly and menacing, '"Bury it in the foundations of the house. You will be *habtam,* a rich man." Hmph.'

'Well, Emar,' I couldn't help but join in, 'Getachew's son was rich, wasn't he?' I looked at her slyly. She turned her head my way, eyes narrowed.

'Until his wife left him, his cows ran away, his foot fell off, and he died, I suppose, yes.' I didn't even try to stop the laughter. 'What good are riches if they come without happiness? The *shagwara* knows nothing of the latter, preoccupied as he is with the former. Idiot man.' As if repeating it made it beyond dispute.

I smiled at the memory as I followed the figures of Indie and my sisters out of Etashy's *sahrbet*. The mourners would take a more direct route to the church, cutting along the side of the sandstone wall that contained the hospital before following the path of the zebu and sheep and goats down to the river, crossing it on a rickety bridge no more than tree trunks laid across it and bound together with vines. It washed out every *keremt,* every rainy season, as the level of the river rose, only to be replaced once again. Once across the river, it was just a short walk up the hill to the graveyard. All around the Church, shaded by eucalyptus, the mourners would wait patiently. It was the time of *ye Fasika tsom,* the fast of Easter, and according to Orthodox tradition, no food, including the funeral feast, could be consumed until the afternoon prayers had finished. The burial could happen though, with crowds of people jostling together, following Etashy's body as it was carried on the shoulders of six men. Heavy stones were passed from hand to hand, until they covered the red soil above her body. Spades, stained the same colour, moved again, adding enough to bring the level of her grave to that of the land. The hyenas wouldn't be able to get to her now, she could rest in peace.

As we walked back to the planks of wood balanced across large rocks that served as benches, women flitted around us, handing out red plastic plates heaped with *injera* and *misr wot*. The feast was shared by all, some going back for seconds, some washing their hands with water collected that morning from the river before entering the church for a moment of contemplation and prayer. I glanced around at my sisters and Indie, raising an eyebrow. A quick shake of the head from Aklila, the eldest and therefore still in charge, despite the fact we were all grown women with children of our own. As I had hoped, she didn't believe we needed to join the mourners in the church, and instead we made our way through the dappled shadows and to the path that would eventually take us back to the village. Mesmora and Raphael had stayed with some of the youngsters at Geremew's *sahrbet*, and I could feel the ache in my breasts that meant Mesmora, at least, would have woken from his lunchtime sleep and would want milk. A quick look at Indie, who touched her own swollen breasts in agreement, told me it would be the same for Raphael. The hours of sleep that came over the boys in the midday, when their little bodies lay curled up next to each other, arms entwined, the breath of one on the hair of the other, was the only time there was ever anything akin to silence in our house. At any other time of the day, it took deliberate effort to make oneself heard. The laughter of Yordannos and Mekdes, as light and tinkling as songbirds, provided the backing soundtrack, with the yells and shouts and giggles of Mesmora and Raphael the unexpected percussion. Indie's happy, teasing chatter was the melody, and my responses the chorus. Interlaced though all of that came the clucking of our chickens, the flapping of laundry drying in the sunshine, the singing of the birds in the *gwaro*, the calling of our cat, Teschew, for her kittens, and, if there was electricity, the music of Ethiopian artists played through crackling speakers. It was a home full of life, there was no doubting that, and I looked forward to leaving the subdued air of the *luxor*.

It would take us less time to walk back than it had to walk here given we were no longer among the crowd of villagers. After taking it in turns to cross the river, holding out hands to help the person behind us, and finding the dusty track into the forest, I glanced to my left through the trees. There was another graveyard here. None of the graves were marked. There were no headstones, no crosses. But it was encircled by a fence of vines braided through upright posts, a construction not unlike the design of the bridge, and all along it, flowering bushes had grown. It was a beautiful, peaceful place, woven into the nature around it in the dappled sunshine, not quite on consecrated ground, but just within the imagined reach of the touch of the church's spiritual protection, at the northernmost end of it. This was the graveyard for those who were Christian in life, but not in death. For suicides and the excommunicated. The graveyard where Alem's husband, Habtu, had been laid to rest just a handful of days previously. Like all those he lay alongside now, he hadn't been allowed the full burial of a Catholic. We hadn't filled the pews of the church, followed behind Alem and her children as they led the procession to the altar, listened to the priest read the final sacrament. Instead, his body was kept in the *sahrbet* he had shared with his family in life, before being carried directly to the graveyard.

As if the church couldn't quite bear to allow him to go on without sharing one last service, though, the priest had still been there. Both in the *sahrbet* where he murmured over the shroud and held his cross to the forehead of Habtu's heartbroken family, and at the graveside, where his voice echoed through the trees, leading the prayers. It had always fascinated me, the burial of the so-called sinners. And for all that I had grown increasingly frustrated, angry even, with Habtu for being unable to fight his fears and cast off the shadows of madness that had taken over him, I did not think him a bad man. He had been a good and kind husband, a doting father, and he deserved peace, salvation, an eternity of Heaven, not of Hell. Yet his actions jarred with what I believed. It was the prerogative of God alone to take a life. But were his failings really those? Were they failings? Were they even his? These were questions I hadn't asked myself whilst he was still alive, incensed as I was for what he was putting Alem and his children through. But now he had died, my guilt had forced me to re-examine what I thought. That started, although I didn't realise it at the time, when Indie commented in passing that she likes the fact that in Amharic the phrase is the same for those with physical illness as for those with mental illness: a woman is *amamat*, a man *amamew.*

It's amazing how much you learn about your own language when teaching it to someone else. When I thought about this, I started to wonder about why. Did we not differentiate because there was no need to do so? Because whether a person has pneumonia or psychosis, neither is by choice? When I forced myself to think of Habtu's last months in this way, I felt the last vestiges of my anger begin to slip. He hadn't chosen what had happened to him, and he hadn't been able to control it, any more than he could control it when he was admitted to hospital with typhoid. And as I realised that, I felt the space left behind by the anger filled with sadness instead.

We had tried everything we could in the weeks leading up to his death, but even the Holy Water splashed over him in ever-generous amounts couldn't drive out the demons. With each day that passed, I couldn't help but feel like we were simply holding off the inevitable. Alem was so tightly wired that even seemingly insignificant moments took on huge meaning, sowing seeds of fear in the spaces of her mind. Simple trips to the *shintebet*, the long drop, were fraught with worry. Had he managed to slip a shard of broken glass up his sleeve without anyone seeing? Would the few moments of privacy he was still accorded behind the flimsy plastic sheeting that made up the walls be all it took? The inexorableness of his death hovered over us all. It is because of that feeling, I think, that when, one afternoon, Alem's youngest son Wasay walked the kilometres from the falling-down hut in the church grounds where Habtu had been kept to the Clinic, telling Alem with tears in his eyes that he had been sent to buy poison for the rats, part of us knew that this was all a smokescreen, a diversion. There were rats, that was true, but there were always rats, and Habtu had never been worried about that before. Wasay was only a child, no more than 10 or 11 Alem thought, and entirely without the scepticism or cynicism that would have made him wonder why Habtu had sent him away. All too aware of what his father had been going through, for Wasay, like his slightly older sister Dirshe and brother Nigusay, had taken his turn watching Habtu in the village, he had known that something was amiss, but believed it to be connected to the poison itself, rather than the time alone that his absence gave Habtu. Alem, older, more sceptical, more cynical, had left straightaway, brushing a hand over Wasay's head, reassuring him he had done the right thing. But as my eyes had met Indie's briefly, the feeling of foreboding was reflected there. And when, no more than an hour later, the phone call we had dreaded for weeks finally came through, I understood that we had started grieving his loss some time ago. The Habtu I knew as a child, the Habtu that Alem had married all those years ago, the Habtu who had tussled with his sons and ticked his daughter, had already left us. Another similarity, then, between a devastating sickness of the body and a debilitating sickness of the mind.

The *luxor* started that afternoon, and would continue for weeks. When Etashy died days later, the procession of women with black gauzy scarves draped over their hands and thrown over one shoulder and men with a hat pulled low over their eyes would cross the *meda* as the mourners made their way from the *sahrbet* of one to the *sahrbet* of the other. Alem and Selam would also visit each other, unable to find any words of comfort, but offering their presence nonetheless, a moment in someone else's grief to escape their own.

It was a few weeks later when, unbidden, Alem was waiting at the gates of the Clinic one morning, dressed in the black of a widow. A generation previously, she would also have proudly shown her bare head, shaved the morning after the death of a family member. It's a tradition that has mostly faded, instead replaced by a black *shajsh*, a scarf, that would cover her hair for the length of the mourning. I was surprised to see her, but when I opened my mouth to reassure her that she needn't come to work yet, I didn't even have the chance to get the words out before she spoke.

'I need to be here, Atsede.'

Nodding, Indie reached a hand out to quieten me before slipping it through the bars of the gates to slide across the lock. She pushed them open, and gestured for Alem to go in. As more time passed after Habtu's death, Alem started to smile again. Often this was at the antics of Mesmora and Raphael, who were getting into more and more mischief every day, but also at the patients who came and the babies who were born. And when Selam came by one morning, asking if Reddit could stay with us while she continued to greet the mourners who had come to pay tribute to the loss of Etashy, Alem gained her own little shadow. Whether Reddit sensed in Alem the same sadness that plagued her mother, or whether she just needed someone to help her stand up to the rambunctious boys, we weren't sure, but every morning she sidled up to Alem, a pudgy hand finding the folds of a long black skirt. With Mesmora and Raphael to distract her, and Reddit demanding affection, the heaviness that had settled over Alem's shoulders started to lift.

One afternoon, the three children were sitting together, as close as they could get without quite being on top of one another. In one hand, they each had a pen, and in the space between them lay an open textbook. Unaware of our ability to see through the crack in the wood, they laughed happily to themselves, taking it in turns to scribble meaninglessly on the paper.

'*Beteratera,*' Mesmora was always the ringleader, giving imperious instructions to Reddit, six months younger, and Raphael, six months younger again. But neither seemed to mind. Mesmora held out the crayon for Raphael to take. Its yellow wax was clearly prized far beyond the dull black ink of the Clinic pens. 'Please, *bey.*' That was Indie's teaching, the insistence on please and thank you. It had been sweet initially, watching the boys make sure that everyone minded their manners. But now not so much as a glass of water could be passed from hand to hand without a chorus of please and thank yous accompanying it. On the occasion that anyone forgot, it was a terrible transgression met with much clicking of a tongue and exaggerated sighs from both Mesmora and Raphael. 'PLEASE, *bey.*' 'Say PLEASE,' they would insist.

I knocked lightly on the door, and Alem called their names, watching as they jumped guiltily. Mesmora quickly grabbed the book and held it behind his back, apparently unaware that, opened up, it was far bigger than he was broad.

'Indie will tell you off, Mesmora. You can't draw on books. What happened to the paper we gave you?' Sheepishly, Mesmora moved to one side, pointing at the pile of shredded bits tucked under the desk. Raphael squatted down, grabbing a handful, laughing, then stood up, throwing it at Reddit, also laughing. Within a moment, the three of them had thrown more and more into the air until it looked like it was snowing, giggling wildly the whole time. Next to me Alem laughed too, a sound I had missed. I heard footsteps behind us, and turned to see who it was. *Ere, tatenkaki jidgewoj,* I thought to myself, *be careful, children.* Indie stepped around us and looked at the chaos inside the birth room, the obstetric textbook lying crookedly on the chair, bright yellow lines scrawled across it, bits of paper floating down and covering the desk, the bed, and the three young children looking up at her with wide smiles, and not the slightest hint of remorse. She turned to Alem and I, wide-eyed and condemning, before looking back to the children.

'Right!' she exclaimed, 'Who did this? I'm going to get you!' Hands raised in claws above her shoulders, she gave a realistic growl and started forward. Screaming in terrified delight, the three of them scattered, darting around us and out into the sunshine, Mesmora and Raphael finding Aster to hide behind while Reddit tucked herself behind Alem. Laughing, Indie turned to us. 'What a mess! I thought they were a little too quiet.' I nodded in agreement, grinning at the naughtiness, while Alem continued to chuckle.

Indie's eyes met mine briefly, flicking to a laughing Alem and back. I nodded ever so slightly, acknowledging the silent message she was sending. Alem was laughing again. It had been weeks since we had heard that sound. Indie's smile softened with relief for a moment, before she spun on her heels, growling again, louder, for the benefit of the three small sets of eyes still fixed on her. She turned away from us, pretending to look under the bench, in through the windows, calling their names all the while.

'Reddit! Moya! Raffy! Where are you? I'm coming to find you!' Stifled giggles rang out before Mesmora gave in, and came out from his hiding place behind Aster, shrieking as he ran across the cobblestones and into the waiting room. Seeing his friend make a dash for it, Raphael followed, a little slower but laughing just as loudly. Reddit, reaching for Alem's hand, pulled her after them, her giggles contagious.

Smiling at them, Indie turned to me. 'Selam is here. She looks tired.' Again, I nodded. I had thought the same thing. The skin under her eyes was bruised, and her usually rounded face seemed more angular. 'Do you think we can help?'

Sighing, I bent to sweep a few of the scraps of paper up. 'I don't think so, Indie. She's just sad. Let her be sad, there's no shame in it. In a little while, when she's ready, she'll be okay again. Is Reddit's bag in here?'

'No, it's on the bench. It's amazing how different Reddit is now, isn't it! So energetic and playful.'

It was true. Reddit was a completely different little girl from the listless, pale, subdued child who had first gone to Addis Ababa more than a month ago. Her life had changed drastically since then, in part for the better, in part not. While her health had, undoubtedly, improved beyond recognition, thanks in no small part to the units of plasma and blood they poured into her tiny veins, not to mention the tiny glass vials of shockingly expensive IgG antibodies, one of which cost almost an entire month's salary. But the death of her grandmother had thrown her family's routine into disarray. Until now, whenever Selam and Kibebe were at work, Reddit and Tensu would go to the village, to stay with Etashy and Amarech for the day. Now Selam wasn't sure what would happen, or whether Amarech, who had given up school, college, employment, any chance at marriage to stay with her mother, would now choose to move away and start her own life. It was this that had brought Reddit to the Clinic. With two children always about, and often three or four if Aster's sons came too, adding another required little adaptation. In any case, Selam's *gowza*, tribe, was Ergah, like me, which made her as close as family, so there was no question we would look after her youngest child when she needed us to.

We finished chasing the last few bits of paper, stacking them neatly in a pile on the chair, ready for tomorrow when, no doubt, the boys would be back to find them once more. Hearing the pattering of feet and the laughter of the three of them running up the veranda, Indie's fierce threats all but forgotten in the face of their new game of chase, we stepped out, looking for Selam. When we found her, she was just outside the gates, leaning against one of the sandstone columns that held it aloft, talking to Seyfu, the older of the

Clinic's guards, who managed to say something entirely irreverent and always entertaining every time we saw him. Judging by Selam's laughter, a welcome change from the strained smile that had become such a familiar expression, this was exactly what had happened. Seyfu turned to us, oversized jacket pulled tight around him, despite the warmth of the sunset, and eyes watering slightly, a leftover from the trachoma that had brought him to the brink of blindness before he was operated on by Dr Solomon, the visiting optometrist who held a monthly surgical programme at the hospital. Slim and wrinkled, we always wondered what would happen if a *laybr,* a thief, ever genuinely made an attempt to break into the Clinic. Watching him break the bread roll he had bought for dinner, and hand half to Selam, I was grateful for his uncomplicated, understated ways, and was reminded, as I always was, of my late uncle in his simple approach to life.

Reddit came up behind me, one hand brushing my leg as she spied her mother.

'Ser!' she called, leaping into her arms, chatting in the incomprehensible but enthusiastic language of a toddler who hasn't quite learnt the words to keep up with their thoughts. I watched the relief spread through Selam's body, emanating from her arms wrapped tightly around her daughter. What a gift a child is, I thought, turning to see my own son balanced on one of Indie's hips, while Raphael was on the other. It was just as well we weren't as slim as eucalyptus, Indie and I had often joked as we lifted our own, or each other's, or both of the boys up. At least they had a place to sit! She moved beside me, Mesmora holding out his hands to come to me as she did so. We talked quietly with Selam for a few minutes before she bade us farewell. With our backs against the blue gate, the sun sinking below the horizon, and our sons in our arms, content for a rare moment to be still, we watched her go, grateful to know she wasn't going to be alone as she continued to be sad, and to miss Etashy, grateful her children would be with her, reminding her of happiness.

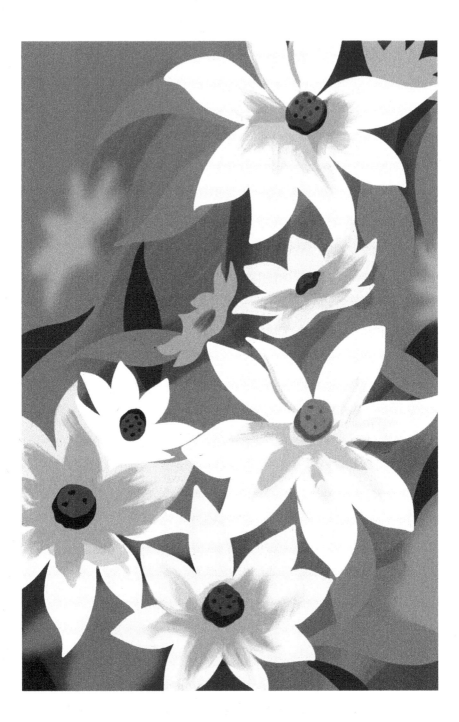

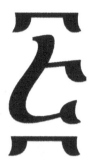

5

Sabrina

Indie

I slipped her tiny, fragile body out of the night swaddling, preparing to check her vital signs, expecting, by her remarkably robust cry of protest, that her breathing, pulse, temperature, and colour would be holding steady. But as the cloth came away from her head and I looked for her fontanelles (the soft dents in the skull bones, one at the front, one the back, which react dramatically either to infection by bulging outwards or to dehydration by sinking inwards), a gasp of horror left me before I could control it. Somehow, in the mere handful of hours between my last check just shy of midnight last night and now, a nasty and seemingly deeply infected wound had opened up. The vicious, yellow pus was pooled right over the fontanelle I had set out to find.

I couldn't believe it, and felt my heart sinking and the pressure of tears behind my eyes. This miracle baby, born weighing just 800g and twelve weeks too soon, the surviving twin who had made it through every day so far, surely couldn't survive such an injury. Her mother, Samira, had seen my reaction and sat up straight, pausing in the middle of her breakfast meal of injera and scrambled eggs, one hand still raised halfway to her mouth. She spoke only Guraginya, and although my command of this tribal dialect was still far from perfect, I couldn't leave her worrying, so I beckoned her to join me at the cotside. After washing her hands under the tap just outside, straightening her dress, and folding the black plastic bag back over the injera that lined it and held her eggs, Samira stood next to me as I tried to explain her daughter now had another, huge challenge to overcome. Samira looked closely at the fine, dark hairs of the little head in front of us, one hand absently caressing Sabrina's side, careful, without even realising it, not to disturb the wires helping to monitor the levels of oxygen in her blood. As I watched sadly, trying to gauge her reaction, wondering how much I had managed to convey, I saw her concern turn slowly to puzzlement before, much to my alarm, a giggle escaped between the fingers she had suddenly clapped over her mouth.

Unsure of how exactly to handle this, but aware too that sometimes the pressures and uncertainties of having a premature baby manifest in unexpected ways, I cast my eyes wildly over the dividing walls into the nurse's station of the surgical ward next door. There, to my relief, was Selam. She had been leaning on the edge of the desk drawing up antibiotics for the women who had had caesarean sections the day before, watching the whole drama unfold, and was now looking on with an expression of barely suppressed amusement at my bewilderment.

'Help me', I half mouthed, half moaned, reverting to Amharic, the language with which I was far more comfortable.

Shaking slightly with silent mirth, Selam carefully put the vial of medication down next to the patient's records, made a quick note that the dose was yet to be given, slipped her pen back into her pocket, and made her way around the low walls and into the makeshift neonatal area. As she came, passing Samira with a whoop of laughter, my confusion mounted. Hardly believing what I was seeing, Selam and Samira had tears of laughter gathering in the corners of their eyes, despite the seriousness of the situation. I now had the slightly panicked air of a clinician who knows something is going very wrong.

'Indie, come here,' it was Selam, surely about to set all of this straight and explain what was going on, 'and look. It's butter'.

'What?'

'It's butter.'

'Butter?'

'Yes.'

'Butter, butter?'

'Yes, Indie, it's butter butter. From milk, from cows. Butter'.

It was a mark of how deeply unsettled I had been just moments before that my first thought on being told there was butter on my patient's head was one of utter relief.

'Selam, why is there butter on her head?'

'Not her head, on her *sumbot,* her fontanelle, to keep her safe, and prevent her from becoming dehydrated.'

It was one of the many traditions around the postnatal period. Even though I had been here for months now, around the babies of patients in the hospital and babies of friends in the villages, this was the first time I had seen it. By now, most of the staff had heard what went on, and had also found some reason to come by the Neonatal Unit, resting elbows on the windowsill and looking through, laughing. At the very least all this glee had to raise Samira's spirits, even if it was at my expense. And, after I'd realised that little Sabrina was not terribly unwell and her mother was not having a mental health crisis, I could see the funny side too. I enjoyed the laughter, all too aware that the moments of light-hearted fun are few and far between when babies born too soon have a steep uphill fight to survive. As Sabrina continued to gain weight, nourished by the love and breastmilk of her mother, a tentative confidence in her ability to survive was growing. I spent more time in the Delivery Room, rather than at her bedside, but often gravitated back to Samira's gentle smile and her daughter's tenacious will to live. I enjoyed sitting with them, watching Sabrina stay awake for a little longer each week, kick a little harder, outgrow the tiny knitted hats.

She was a thread of hope woven into the cloth of the hospital, and as I sat around the table with the Sisters in the evenings, I was asked about her. My answers were often followed by their own stories of the remarkable survival of patients over the decades since the hospital first opened its doors. I spent a little over a year living in the convent at the end of the path leading away from the hospital, shaded by trees. Whilst I spent the most time with Dr Rita, calmed by her unshakeable acceptance of everything faced in her role as the obstetrician, and Dr Toni, whose irreverent humour and take-no-prisoners attitude often reduced me to tears of laughter, dinner brought all of the Medical Missionary Sisters together, so I had the chance to get to know them all. Tiny, ancient Sr Inge, whose voice wavered as she spoke, and hands shook as she held her daily mug of *birtukan,* orange juice, but who remembers the first days of the hospital, when patients were treated in one of just two rooms, and supplies were bought down from Addis Ababa on a donkey. Statuesque Sr Elise, who, despite thirty years in Ethiopia, still wore the beautiful salwar kameez of her Indian homeland, and laughed a deep, infectious laugh when admitting she did so even in her role as a midwife all those years ago, when the guards would keep watch over the women through the night, only calling her when they saw the women sweat because not long after, they would also see the women birth, they said. Sr Carol and Sr Elaine, the American nuns who could not have been more different physically, the first short and slim, the second decidedly not, but who held nostalgic conversations about their homes in the States that none of the rest of us could follow. Sr Florence, the teasing, merry Ghanaian who had travelled to Ethiopia to spend time learning more deeply about the service of the Medical Missionary Sisters in Africa. The final four chairs at the table were filled with Ethiopians, Sr Nigist and Sr Belaynesh, the youngest of the Sisters, still in their fifties but decades younger than their companions who were in their seventies and eighties, who oversaw the children's nursing and the administration respectively, and the two girls just starting their journey into the Order, the novitiates, Ayane and Birkenesh.

For the most part, the Sisters' lives together were harmonious, dedicated to serving God through serving the sick and destitute. But, as Atsede was quick to point out, they were also simply women, and it was inevitable that with so much time spent in such close quarters, friction sometimes arose. And when it did, without the chance to spend any real length of time apart to let it pass, resentment simmered under the surface for weeks. With their places in all the positions of leadership within the functioning of the hospital, from Dr Rita as the Medical Director to Sr Belaynesh as the Administrative Director, it also meant the difficulties in the hospital followed the Sisters to the convent. I was in an unusual position, having formed close relationships with so many of the midwives with whom I spent so much time, but also living with the Sisters and developing friendships with each of them.

It only became apparent that I would ever have to choose where my loyalties lay when I found myself caught up in the midst of a conflict. Sitting one night with Dr Rita as we awaited a referral from a distant health centre, I had spoken to her of my frustrations at what was happening between one of the Sisters and the staff, particularly Atsede. A little undiplomatically perhaps, given the bonds of purpose she shared with the Sisters, as Dr Rita and I spoke,

I had railed against some of the decisions that had been made, and also how I had been treated when I had made it clear that I would stand with Atsede. Dr Rita, ever thoughtful, turned to me and told me that one's behaviour reflected little of the world or the circumstances, but much of one's own self. And, as such, it is the responsibility of each individual to recognise their shortcomings, and find a way to overcome them. It wasn't a reprimand, I didn't think, and the hand she laid on my arm as I looked at her with knitted eyebrows confirmed that. But it made me think.

Perhaps her ability to truly live by this, and refrain from becoming involved in bickering, was a result of living in such close proximity with the women in the convent, where she had no choice but to learn to tolerate them. There is little true privacy as a missionary nun, I came to see, with so much time spent together and every movement known, and the real lesson I took from my year with the Medical Missionary Sisters is the value of respecting the sanctity of a person's mind.

The Sisters, for the most part, tread lightly with each other's thoughts, shying away from intervening in private problems unless they are asked. There are exceptions, of course, but I learnt much about patience and forbearance from the difficulties that arose following a breakdown in my relationship with one of the Sisters. And as she had that first night, when we sat waiting for the referral, Dr Rita continued to quietly make herself available but hesitated to step in. It was on me, and on Atsede, my close friendship with whom was responsible for my involvement in the first place, to decide on our own courses of action and to behave accordingly. While this was difficult at the time, looking back now I appreciate the value of what I learnt in having to construct our own means of coping with challenges.

In any case, the days spent in the Delivery Room were so varied and so interesting that it left little time to dwell on the convoluted nature of human relationships. As my confidence in my own clinical abilities and language skills grew, helped along in no small part by the gentle guidance of Atsede and Selam, I spent more and more time there, staying late into the evenings and through the weekends. Unlike the first few months of my time as a midwife here, I now understood the flow of the Delivery Room, no longer needed translators, and knew I could appropriately and safely manage most of what I was likely to see. Every month, along with hundreds of straightforward births, I was also exposed to different and often rare obstetric situations. Working alongside clinicians as experienced as Dr Rita and Atsede was an incredible opportunity, and I was determined to make the most of it, just as happy to be assisting the surgeons as they performed caesareans, hands stretched out to pass over instruments, as standing with a woman, hands stretched out to catch her baby. The days passed quickly, but almost every one held the promise of the unexpected.

After checking that I wasn't needed, and whispering quickly to Sabrina that I was very pleased it was only butter on her fontanelle, I smiled at Atsede, slipping my arm through hers and wandering back to the Delivery Room. As we passed through the first set of doors, Atsede was quickly hailed by the relatives of a woman who had birthed in the night, while I found myself being forcefully steered by Selam towards the obstetric operating theatres, where, she informed me, Dr Rita had already started operating. Smiling at that, unsurprised that Dr Rita, who had been known to anaesthetise, operate on, and see a woman through recovery single-handed if the situation required it, I donned the plastic apron and white clogs Selam was holding out and allowed myself to be chivvied along ahead of her. Standing at the scrub sinks while Selam paused, turning to Atsede as she called out, 'Indie and I are going in with Asnakech and the twins', I remembered the operation a few evenings earlier, when the electricity had cut out, as it so often does, and we had to scramble to find the torches stored on the windowsill. Unperturbed by being plunged into sudden darkness, when we flicked the lights on, holding the torches steady to direct the beams of light towards the operating table, we saw Dr Rita hadn't even paused in her suturing, simply moving by touch rather than sight. I had asked her about it, my voice tinged in equal parts with awe and apprehension.

'*Ayoo* Indie,' she replied – she too had picked up the expressions of the Gurage – 'How many times have I operated through the darkness? It is much better now there are torches. Thirty years ago, we had only candles. Can you imagine? All it took was a gust of air, and they went out.'

'Thirty years ago. There can't have been spinal anaesthesia thirty years ago?' I knew there wasn't, having spoken to Solomon about its introduction at the hospital a decade later. 'What did you use?'

'We soaked a cloth in ether anaesthesia, and held it over the nose and mouth of the women.'

I shook my head in disbelief, finding it hard to believe the circumstances under which Dr Rita had worked. Then I slowly realised something else. 'Hang on, Dr Rita, you used open ether anaesthesia at one end, and a candle at the other? Oh, my God!'

Ruefully, she shook her head. 'I know. I sometimes can't believe that we all survived. But there was never a fire, and we just had to be very careful about where we put the candles.' I watched her in amazement.

Half an hour later, in the middle of writing up the notes, I was still smiling as I recorded the details of the three girls Dr Rita had lifted from their mother's womb, remembering their warm, soft bodies, and angry cries of protest at being separated from each other. As soon as Selam and I had dried and dressed them, the tiny sisters had curled around each other, limbs entwined, seeking the closeness they'd shared while carried by their mother. The third baby had come of something of a surprise, given we were only expecting twins, but after Dr Rita's distinctive laugh rang out across the theatre upon the discovery of another girl, tucked away behind her sisters, I had managed to find another cloth and spin quickly back into the room to collect her. When together, they had settled almost straight away, waiting patiently for their first feed. It would come soon enough, after Dr Rita and Naty had finished the operation.

Her newest daughters brought the number of children Asnakech had to eight, and given that this pregnancy had been complicated by the beginning of a dehiscence of the scar left by her previous caesarean, she had agreed that BTL, bi tubal ligation, could be performed. This meant that, after tying the delicate filament of suture around her uterine tubes, Naty would remove a section of them, interrupting the path used by her eggs to make their way down the tubes into the uterus, and so preventing another pregnancy. Asnakech had then been taken to the surgical ward to recover, where Selam and I, arms full of her daughters, had, a few minutes earlier, found her eldest daughter and youngest sister, who were the same age and rarely seen apart, waiting impatiently to meet the new girls. Delighted smiles had lit up the faces of the young women as they laid claim to a baby each, and then bickered good-naturedly over who would also hold the third. Selam and I had joined in, laughing at the antics of the affectionate family the babies were lucky enough to be joining.

Heading back to the Delivery Room, we had nearly collided with Dr Rita. With hardly a moment to take off her operating gown and shoes, she had been met at the theatre doors by a flustered looking Gete, asking that she come quickly to gynaecological outpatients with Naty, the student surgeon, as there was a woman who needed to be seen urgently. I caught Naty's eye and grinned at him, remembering the surgery the day before, and the many times we had told the story of it since, including during the last caesarean that evening.

'And then,' Belete had said as he deftly manoeuvred the uterus back into the woman's abdomen after suturing the incision with his precise, neat stitches, 'I heard Natnael actually hiss at Indie, telling her to not react but go to him that instant'.

Solomon, the anaesthetist, was laughing quietly as he listened to Belete telling the tale, one hand resting reassuringly on the braided hair of the woman in front of him, who was also listening intently. 'Isn't that right?' Belete looked at me.

'Oh, yes,' I picked up the thread of his story. 'So, I edged around the table, trying not to distract Dr Rita, and there, would you believe, were these two skinny legs sticking out from beneath the gown!' The laughter continued, and I could see even Natnael was grinning reluctantly beneath his mask. 'I couldn't work out what I was seeing at first, until I saw the green trousers in a puddle on the floor.'

'Did Dr Rita not realise?' Solomon asked. Dr Rita didn't have a reputation for seriousness, not like Dr Abdulsemed, the general surgeon, but she was so respected that the thought of her knowing about Naty's trousers falling down was enough to cause great embarrassment.

'I think she might have, especially given Naty had then tried to stop them falling by spreading his legs as wide as he could, before accepting it wasn't going to work.' The skin now sutured too, Belete and Naty had wiped iodine across the wound before carefully pressing a length of gauze over it, Belete laughing all the while, and the look in Naty's eyes was something between amusement and exasperation.

I could see, now, as we waited for Dr Rita, a similar look as Naty realised exactly what I was thinking. He narrowed his eyes in my direction, and shoved against me gently before standing to attention as Dr Rita turned to us.

'Notes are on the desk, can you write them up please, Indie? You've got the baby details anyway, haven't you?' I smiled and nodded my agreement. The weights were written on the glove I'd been wearing as I reached out to take the last of the babies, then promptly thrown into the theatre buckets after wrapping her warmly in a fleecy blanket, completely forgetting the three little numbers scribbled quickly onto the back of my hand. I turned to Selam at exactly the same time as she turned to me.

'The gloves!' The realisation had come at the same time. Selam, laughing, had ushered me off in the direction of the theatres, before making her own way back to the Delivery Room. By the time I'd finished tentatively picking gloves and gauze out of the bucket at the foot of the operating table, and let out a whoop of success at having found the missing glove, complete with all the times and weights, and pushed through the swing doors back into Delivery, both Selam and Atsede were busy with women, the plaid curtains pulled closed around bed spaces, and quiet voices explaining what they could expect to happen. Glancing to the desk, I saw where

Lubaba, the tiny, vivacious woman in charge of cleaning the theatres, had left Asnakech's notes, and settled into the chair to write.

I'd just about finished by the time I heard Atsede's voice call out. I paused, looking up at her as she walked over. She seemed preoccupied, anxious even, though I couldn't understand why. I leaned to look through the curtain at the bedspace she had just come from and smiled, recognising the sweet, round face of Maregnesh, Atsede's childhood friend.

'Okay.' Still unable to reconcile the concern written into every line of Atsede's expression with Maregnesh lying calmly on the bed, I asked 'What's going on? What do you need?'

It was unusual to see Atsede so uncertain. When the storms raged around her, Atsede was unflappably calm, focused and controlled, knowing, instinctively, the next step. She must have come from a line of midwives, Dr Rita had said of her once. And yet, here she was, hands twisting the pinards held there, chewing her bottom lip. I shifted in my chair, turning to face her.

'Okay. What do you want me to do? Shall I ask Dr Rita to come and assess?'

I wasn't even sure if Atsede had heard me. Her eyes were unfocused, looking into the distance, as the pinard continued to twirl round and round in her hands. It made me dizzy just looking at it. Feeling unnerved now, I opened my mouth to ask again. Before I could though, Atsede blinked, then looked at me, nodding.

Shaking my head in confusion, I stood up, and pushed aside the chairs that had been moved in front of the open doorway to stop impatient relatives coming into the midwives' area. Smiling a greeting at the women in the room on the other side, and waving off an offer of *kawa*, I wondered where Dr Rita would be. Walking the length of the veranda, the backbone of the hospital, I glanced either side of me, looking through the open windows of the Surgical Ward and the Medical Ward to my left, and the Operating Theatres and Neonatal Unit to my right. She wasn't there. Sighing, I continued along, passing nurses with arms full of notes, and visitors with woven bags holding food for those admitted. In the obstetrics and gynaecology outpatients' room, I found her at last. Hesitant to interrupt, I could see from her movements that she was about to scan a woman whose vast abdomen hung pendulously in front of her. Twins? I wondered to myself in passing. But then I remembered Atsede's agitation and took a deep breath.

'Dr Rita? I'm sorry to interrupt. But would you come with me please?' I smiled apologetically at the woman.

'Indie, I'm just about to scan.' I was right. 'Is this necessary?'

'Yes, Dr Rita, I think so. Atsede has a woman she wants you to see. She's…' I paused as I struggled to find the right words to describe it. '…on edge.'

Dr Rita looked at me curiously, head cocked to one side. 'On edge?' A smile crossed her features before it faded into a look of vague alarm. 'Atsede, on edge. Let's go.'

Grateful, I stepped out of the room ahead of her, Dr Rita calling instructions to Admasu, the wonderful IESO surgeon who served as her right hand, just behind me. As we walked swiftly back down the slope towards the inpatient wards, Dr Rita asked me more. She led the way to the left, past the administration rooms and on to the veranda that ran along the outside of the hospital, lined by tall trees and flowering bushes. It wasn't the usual way to go, despite the door that opened up to the walkway from the sluice serving the Delivery Room.

'I won't get asked to stop to see someone else, this way.' Dr Rita explained, seeing my pace slow down slightly as she took the turn. Nodding in understanding, I continued my explanations.

'I'm not entirely sure what's happening, really. It's Maregnesh, a friend of Atsede's from Sisa. First baby, full term, easy pregnancy. She was lying on the bed when I last saw her, conscious and talking. All her vitals were fine. I don't think she had contractions. But Atsede is very anxious something is wrong.' It wasn't much by way of a handover, or a clarification, and I felt a little silly having taken Dr Rita away from her work without a clear reason as to why. But then the image of Atsede's restless hands came to mind. 'Yes, something is wrong.'

Dr Rita pushed open the door in front of us, and moved down

the length of the Delivery Room, passing bedspaces with curtains pulled closed until she came to Atsede at the end. She nodded in greeting. I followed her, staying quiet until I could catch Atsede's eyes, then made my way back to the desk, where I could finish the last few notes from the operation before handing it over to the nurses on the Surgical Ward. As I wrote, I watched Dr Rita come through the curtains, my eyes following her as she moved the old ultrasound machine stored in the corner to the bedside. A moment later, I heard a sharp intake of breath. Atsede wrenched back the curtains, her eyes finding me.

'Abruption. Almost complete. CS, now.' Her eyes were huge, and she was paler than I had ever seen her.

'Oh, my God. Okay.' We looked at each other for a moment before springing into action, gathering everything needed. Atsede had grabbed a cannula and bag of fluid, returning to Maregnesh before I even had time to blink.

'Catheter', I muttered to myself, 'Antibiotics, anaesthetics, prepare for resuscitation, prepare for blood.'

Passing things through to Atsede, I called to Lubaba to fetch Solomon, the anaesthetist, before rushing to the cot kept just outside the operating theatre, where babies who needed resuscitation were taken. With an almost complete abruption, it was remarkable, unbelievable, that Maregnesh's baby was still alive. As I spread a clean white sheet across the cot, lying the bag-valve-mask on top of it, I felt Dr Rita brush past me.

'Back into theatre then, Indie.' Dr Rita said, smiling ruefully as she pulled on an apron and cap before turning to the sinks, 'scrub in, please. You're assisting. Now. Selam is almost finished giving the magnesium sulphate, so she'll take the baby. We don't have time to wait for someone to go and get Admasu.'

I nodded, feeling the adrenaline move through my veins as my hands started to shake slightly. Behind Dr Rita, Maregnesh was walking gingerly towards the operating theatre, Atsede at her side, gripping her elbow tightly and talking in a low, reassuring voice. My heart went out to Maregnesh: with everything changing so quickly, she barely had time to hear an explanation, let alone understand it. But with an abruption, every second mattered, not only for the baby, but also for Maregnesh, who would rapidly be losing blood into her uterus. I sent a silent thanks to whatever it was watching over the hospital that Maregnesh's waters were still intact. At least with that barrier in place, containing the blood, there could only be so much lost. Still, I shuddered, knowing the deceptively capacious space that would have been filling, all morning, with the blood Maregnesh's body was moving into it, half a litre a minute through the huge uterine arteries.

A minute later, with Solomon standing at Maregnesh's head, Dr Rita splashed iodine on her exposed abdomen and began to operate. I couldn't contain the gasp that left me as I saw the litres of blood spilling out of the incision Dr Rita had made through her uterine muscles. My hand on the retractor that was holding her now empty bladder out of the way was covered, and I felt the warm liquid soak through my dress, not quite covered by the plastic apron worn beneath the sterile gown, and drip into my shoes. Dr Rita looked up briefly, concern in her eyes, the only part of her face visible, as her hands, submerged, continued to move, trying to find the baby and bring him safely out. The theatre was absolutely silent, save for the beeping of the machine monitoring Maregnesh's pulse, and the steady whoosh of Solomon pushing air from the bag through the mask into Maregnesh's lungs as he ventilated her, as Dr Rita withdrew her hands and the baby emerged. As soon as he felt the cold air, he cried, an angry declaration of shock. It took a moment for anyone to realise that this baby was alive. I saw Atsede, and Selam a moment later as she came through the door, still pulling on gloves, go limp with relief, as Solomon's low voice began a fervent prayer of thanks, a Guraginya chant that rose as naturally to the lips of the Christians as air. He knew Maregnesh too, having grown up in the same village.

Dr Rita, after placing the wriggling baby into Selam's waiting hands, uttering a 'Thank God', of her own, turned back to Maregnesh, her expression grim. With the suction on, I held it in the uterus, siphoning out as much as I could, watching with trepidation as the amount in the glass jar increased and increased. 3,000ml of blood. Almost half of her circulating volume. Even accounting for amniotic fluid that was mixed with it, it was a huge blood loss. Dr Rita's hands moved quickly, clamping bleeding vessels, repairing the incision. With the muscles stitched together, her hands went around Maregnesh's now empty uterus, pressing together hard, assisting the natural process of contraction with her own efforts. I glanced at the monitoring screen: her blood pressure and pulse were still holding steady. I shook my head as I found Solomon's eyes, nodding to the blood that soaked the operating drapes, spreading in puddles on the floor. He raised his shoulders slightly, echoing my feelings of incredulity.

Maregnesh stayed on the operating table after Dr Rita had finished the operation and stepped away. Atsede and Selam kept vigil, covering her with blankets and pulling the overhead operating lights as close to her body as they could, hoping the heat the bulbs generated would infiltrate through. Keeping her warm was essential now, if her body was to produce the clotting factors needed to prevent further bleeding. As soon as we had showered and changed our clothes, Dr Rita and I found a free bed in the postnatal room, and I lay down as the sting of a needle pricked the crook of my arm. Clenching and releasing my first, watching as my blood flowed into the bag that would soon be hung up at Maregnesh's side, I asked Dr Rita about her vital signs, how they had held steady through all that blood loss.

'Women are remarkable,' came her only answer. I smiled in agreement, taking the small ball of cotton wool Dr Rita held out to me, and pressing it over the tiny hole left by the cannula.

Maregnesh's extraordinary survival, like Samira's, stayed with us, providing a buoyant platform of hope to lean back on even in the midst of the sadness that followed after tragedy the next time it struck. Through the desolation that was to come, I heard Atsede's voice reminding me that it as was important to remember the times when we were there, just in time, with just the right way to help, as it was to remember the times we weren't, and that both carried invaluable lessons. It was a mantra I would keep in my mind as Meske deteriorated.

She needed a team of specialists, an ITU equipped with cutting edge technology, drugs and machines that could take over and support her organs until she healed. Not me, sitting with a blood pressure cuff, an oxygen concentrator, and just three precious vials of the anti-hypertensive drug hydralazine. Before too long, battling the inexorable climb in the blood pressure of a deteriorating body desperately trying to keep cardiac output at life-preserving levels, I ran out of even that. Not ready to lose the futile war to bring her vital signs back to something resembling normal, I needed more medications. It was with a firm gentleness that Dr Rita had shaken her head at my requests, sad but certain. 'It won't save her, Indie. Nothing will save her now. We have to keep it for patients it can help.'

Unable to let go, unwilling to lose another woman, I couldn't turn and walk away empty-handed. 'But maybe if we can control this, we can find more blood to replace what she's lost, we can correct the DIC, get her kidneys working again, stop the acidosis, reverse the damage.' In my frantic mind, stabilising her blood pressure was inextricably linked with her surviving.

'She's dying, Indie'. It was the cool touch of Atsede's hand on my arm that broke through my tunnelled concentration focused in on just her blood pressure, incapable of seeing the full scene playing out. A look passed between her and Dr Rita, one I couldn't decipher, but it spoke of experience and understanding and acceptance. They had been here before, seen this before, teetered on the knife edge between life and death. A nod from Dr Rita, and she turned back to the theatres, leaving me, eyes filling with tears, to Atsede's firm kindness. 'See this through, Indie. Take your seat at your patient's side, and see this through. You are a midwife; this is part of what we must do. We are there for women at their most vulnerable, when they are fierce and when they are frightened. Midwives are guides and guards, and she needs both now more than ever. Don't think of her broken body, think of her untarnished soul. Do your duty, and help her to die with dignity and peace.'

I closed my eyes, and listened to the thrum of the hospital around me. The footsteps of nurses moving between wards, the far-off beeps of machines monitoring the operation Dr Rita was now performing, a mother chiding her daughter, the branches creaking in the winds, calling birds, background conversations, punctuated by laughter and cries and prayers. Gathering my courage, trying to muster something of Atsede's composure, I turned, ready to sit by my dying patient.

It could have been hours later, or minutes, when Meske took her final breath. As I watched her sister accept the finality of Meske's death, a wave of sadness washed over me, followed quickly by frustration. I couldn't understand the unnecessary nature of it all. In another time, in another place, she wouldn't have died. Leaning close to remove the oxygen lines from her nose, the first step in preparing her body for burial, an act which can't be left for too long in the heat of the Ethiopian day, I quietly apologised, deeply regretting that we weren't able to save her.

Standing side-by-side with the nurses of the surgical ward, I touched Meske for the last time, holding her hand as it started to cool, as the nurses washed her body. While her daughters couldn't bring themselves to be there, instead starting the ululating cries of *luxor*, her mother sat, dry-eyed and silent, in the same place she had sat all day. She watched as we prepared her daughter for burial, completely still, as if carved from stone, not moving until her sons lifted Meske's palanquin onto their shoulders, and walked solemnly through the hospital and out across the *meda,* the grasslands, to their village.

Meske would stay in my mind in the years to come. Walking behind Meske's procession, I was struck by the impermanence not only of life, but of all we experience within it. Nothing stays the same, nothing is guaranteed. It takes only one act, one moment, for everything to change irrevocably. Sometimes this is for the better, but sometimes it isn't, and there's no way of knowing which it will be until it has happened.

Not wanting, yet, to return to the Delivery Room to break the news to Dr Rita, I found myself tracing a familiar path to Sabrina's bedside. She had changed hugely in the last month, with little creases starting to form on her legs and arms, an indication of the fat her body was now able to lay down as insurance against future difficulties. Her eyes no longer seemed so prominent in her face, and she had started to wear the little knitted cardigans we had found for her in the cupboards of the Neonatal Unit. She was sleeping peacefully now, a patchwork blanket crocheted from hues of blue and green covering her, one arm tucked at her side, the other resting by her head. I sat heavily on the low cot beside her, sighing and playing with a thread from the blanket. Samira had been watching me closely from her chair by the open window, a place where she could sit to watch everything happening along the veranda outside, but still reach out a hand to calm her baby if needed, and I heard her click her tongue, a sound of sorrow and disbelief often heard in response to a death. She, along with all the patients on the Surgical Ward, had watched as events unfolded around Meske. There was as little privacy in death as there was in birth in a hospital with two patients to a bed, and more than fifty beds in a ward.

Samira shifted in the chair and stood up, crossing the tiled floor to sit next to me. Taking my hand in hers, and settling it on her lap, we sat in silence, remembering Meske. Long before we ever developed a spoken language, humans communicated through their bodies alone. Sitting, now, with Samira, I understood that on a profound level. Sharing the sorrow of death with Samira, who had so recently walked the gamut herself and survived, just through the feeling of her hand in mine, somehow lessened the sadness I carried because we couldn't save her. We sat like that for a while, until I felt able to make my way back to the Delivery Room, ready to feel the promise of new life casting off the memory of death.

'Indie… Indie!' It was a whispering voice full of laughter. I leant back around the curtain, my hand still on the swell of Filseta's abdomen, measuring the length and strength of her contractions.

'Selam, I'm busy. What is it?' I raised an eyebrow at her. Selam hadn't been there during the day, instead taking over as the senior on the night shift, but had heard, as everyone in the villages had, that a woman had died in childbirth that morning. The moment she walked through the doors, Selam had sought out Atsede and me, to ask what happened and give tight hugs when she saw our sadness. It was a sadness I still felt, hours later, when Selam's voice came through the curtains, but with more women coming into the Delivery Room throughout the day, and more babies to welcome into the world, it was tempered now, with the balance of happiness felt when guiding a woman through a birth safely.

Neither of us wanting to go to our respective homes, where we would sit, alone, and think about Meske, Atsede and I had both asked to stay into the evening. Dr Rita, with understanding in her eyes, had agreed, so when Filseta came slowly through the doors, bent at the waist, one hand on her back, it was into my care that she came. This was Filseta's fourth baby, and things were moving fast. She had arrived just a few minutes ago, but her breathing and movements suggested there wouldn't be that much time. She was in good spirits though, with the look of someone who knew what was to come and was keen to get through the pain and finally hold her baby.

'I know. But this is very important. Very serious. I need you to come'. Her words failed to match the tone of poorly concealed delight in her voice, and I could see the mirth in her eyes. Her lips were pressed together in an attempt to suppress a smile, and once she saw my interest was piqued, she reached a hand out, beckoning.

'Filse, I'm going to find my favourite midwife to look after you, and I will be back as soon as I can be.' I didn't really want to leave, I wasn't sure I'd be able to find the same happiness in whatever it was that had Selam smiling, but I knew Atsede would keep an eye on everything with Filseta, and I was already grateful that Selam was trying to keep me from being too sad. I nodded to Selam, and she turned, heading to the scrub sink by the operating theatre to wait. I found Atsede sitting with one of the women, Betsalot, who had given birth earlier that day, a cousin of hers, drinking a small cup of *kawa*, and passing around handfuls of *kollo*, roasted barley. After extracting a promise that Filseta would be in good hands, I shrugged off my white gown, made sure all the notes and boards were up-to-date, and headed off to find Selam.

'Come on, come on, come on! You are so slow!' Now she had my attention, Selam wasted no time in ushering me through the door.

'Selam, let me wash my hands at least, and what is going on?'

'Wait. You'll see. But come on!'

Bemused, but starting to get swept up in her enthusiasm, I let myself be dragged along the hospital's central walkway. It was the start of the night shift, the fourth of seven for Selam, and bitterly cold outside. The torrential rains had started earlier in the afternoon, and it felt as though they would never stop. The water thundered down on the corrugated iron roof, cascading off the trees, the endless soundtrack of the *keremt* wet season. Above us, the skies were black, with no stars shining through and no hint of a moon, the darkness broken only occasionally by lightning streaking across the sky. It was no night to be outside, or travelling to a hospital through knee-deep mud to give birth. And yet, with no other choice, still the women would come.

We reached the end of the walkway and turned towards the Emergency Room. It was long and low, tiled for the most part, but these were old now, chipped and worn. There was a peeling red cross painted over the doorway, muffled voices coming from inside, and a donkey tied at the entrance. I stopped short at that.

'Selam.'

'I know!'

Livestock in the streets or on paths was a common sight. The zebu, goats, and fat-tail sheep made the most of the grasses growing in any unused space. But a donkey tied up in the hospital was unexpected. The rain dripped from the donkey's long ears, and his wet coat lay plastered against him, defining ribs and hip bones. He snorted as we approached, a cloud of air billowing into the night.

'Did you bring me to see a donkey, Selam?' I couldn't keep the teasing out of my voice, glancing at her and grinning, the heaviness that had been sitting over me for the last few hours starting to be dispelled in the comfort of friendship.

She looked back with eyes narrowed, trying to look contemptuous but betrayed by the smile playing around her lips. 'Shut up, and come on.'

We side-stepped the donkey, and still looking at Selam with a perplexed smile, nonetheless I followed her through the always open door.

'Selam, are you bringing everyone to see me? Why? You are a terrible friend. I will be telling your mother.' It was said with mock exasperation, accompanied by a dramatic flinging of his hand back over his eyes. But I could hear the warmth in his voice, and knew the teasing marked the deep affection between these two. They had grown up together, been through school together, seen each other through all the big moments of life. From the same *gowza*, the same tribe, they could never have married, but that didn't lessen the strength of their bond.

'*Aihee*, Naty, stop it. You'll get blood on us!'

Pulling a face at Selam, Naty turned to me, smiling.

'The donkey bit me.'

'The donkey bit him.'

It was said at almost exactly the same time. With a smirk from Selam, and a grimace from Naty.

'Ah, I'm sorry, Naty, that must have really hurt. They have big teeth, those donkeys'. My eyes roamed his arms and legs, looking for a tell-tale bandage. There was no blood on his face, so it couldn't have been there. But his trousers were soaked in it, and a darkened strain spread across both the sleeves of his green jumper. 'Did, ah, you need stitches?' I was still trying to work out why I was here. Dosed up on strong analgesics, Naty didn't come across as particularly distressed by the pain. Watching him more closely, there seemed a sheepish, indignant air about him.

'Yes, to try and stop the blood. I'm going up to Addis though, once the ambulance gets here.'

That confused me. He was stable, conscious, talking. If the surgical intern on duty tonight had already stemmed the bleeding and repaired the wound, why would he need further interventions in Addis Ababa? It took hours to get there, even more so in the middle of the night in the middle of a storm. And it would take him away from his home and his family, something not to be taken lightly. I felt a creeping suspicion tickle the back of my mind and comprehension started to dawn that I was missing something significant.

'Naty.'

'Mm?'

'So, where exactly did the donkey bite you?'

There was a suppressed giggle from Selam, and Naty cast her a withering look.

'Ah'. A pause, and the sheepish expression returned. 'Let me tell you how it happened. I had been at the house of a friend, celebrating their new job. We had beer and *arakay* and *qat*. Probably too much. When I was walking home, I needed to pee. You can see what it's like outside, it's so dark and there's so much rain, but I could make out the shape of bushes and trees up ahead, you know, the ones by the army barracks? I was so relieved! So I, you know, got ready to pee. The drinking had made me a bit unsteady, so I reached out for support against the tree. But then the tree moved. Suddenly. And before I knew it, the tree had become a donkey. Which swung its head round. And bit whatever was in its way. Which just happened to be... well... me. The part of me that was peeing.'

It took me a moment to understand, but then suddenly Selam's amusement fell into place.

'The donkey bit off your penis?

'Yes, the donkey bit off my penis.'

That certainly explained the blood stains on his trousers. But somehow, with a stroke of unbelievable good fortune, the donkey had managed not to bite off any of the delicate central structures, the urethra, or the main blood vessels running through and supplying essential blood. Instead, it was largely a flesh wound, so to speak. And it was likely that there would be no impairment of the normal physiology or function, just scarring and some deformation. Still, it must have hurt. I was amazed Naty remained in such good spirits, and could already understand how his unusual injury had caused so much amusement. I was fully prepared to chide Selam for her insensitivity, but seeing Naty give in and join her laughter, I was reminded once more of the power of humour in coping with adversity. So I smiled back at them.

We sat with Naty for a little longer, until the tell-tale lights of the ambulance bounced across the cobblestones, glittering through the deluge. With bandages packed in place, and words of encouragement uttered, I stood, leaning against the wall, watching Selam help him into the ambulance. There was a team awaiting him in Addis Ababa, a leading urologist and visiting plastic surgeon who, between them, would be far better able to repair the wound. Over the laughter of Selam and Naty, I could hear the donkey snorting behind me, and turned to watch him, wondering once again why he was there at all. Selam smiled at me as she slipped back under the protection of the corrugated iron roof.

'So, there you go. Can you imagine that. Poor Naty.'

'Oh yes, and such sympathy from you! The doctors in Addis Ababa will take good care of him. But Selam, why is the donkey here?'

Her eyes lit up again, and I could see she had been waiting for me to ask just that.

'That Naty. He wanted the surgeons to cut in and get it out! Then sew everything back together. 'You can cut out a baby', he said, 'why can't you cut out the rest of my penis!' Would you believe that? He just refused to come to the hospital without it.'

I joined her laughter, the sound of it echoing off the empty corridors as we walked back to the Delivery Room. I felt Selam's arm come around my shoulder as she pulled me close.

'I'm sorry about your patient, Indie.'

'Meske,' I said, 'Her name was Meske.'

'Meske. It's a terrible thing for a woman to die in childbirth.' Selam kept her arm in place as I smiled at her sadly. 'But it's not great to have your penis bitten off by a donkey, either!'

Without realising, I was chuckling along with her. Her voice softened as she looked at me. 'Keep smiling, Indie. We must not stop happiness from coming. It would be an insult to Meske's memory if all that is left of her is sadness.'

I nodded in agreement, hugging her back, as grateful for her guidance through the challenges as her joy in the successes of everything we see and everything we do as members of this remarkable profession. Together, we walked back to the Delivery Room. Stepping into the dimly lit room, I heard the unmistakable sounds of a woman close to birth, and realised it must be Filseta. Delighted to have made it for the last minutes before her baby was born, I nodded to the curtains pulled closed.

'Selam, that's Filseta. I'll be back in a moment, okay?' She smiled and shooed me in the direction of the groans.

Approaching the curtains, I could hear Filseta's heavy breathing as the contraction waned, and moved a little towards the opening.

'Atse? Filse? I'm back. Can I come in?' I heard a groan in response from Filseta, and, not wanting to disturb the focus she would need to bring her baby into the world, took that as a yes. Gently moving the curtains aside, I stepped through them, eyes at first going to Filseta, whose head was resting on her hand clenched in front of her, before seeing Atsede at her knees. It took me a moment to work out what I was looking at, the contorted angle of Atsede's arms, the floppy white glove dangling from her fingers on one hand, the strangely shaped glove on the other. But as it fell into place, I felt the laughter bubbling up, and clamped a hand over my mouth. She must have tried to get the gloves on in a hurry, misjudging where the holes for her fingers were on one, and failing to get the second one on altogether before reaching out to support the top of the head visible between Filseta's legs. As much as I longed to tease her about this straight away, I knew it would interrupt the peace that Filseta had found, and consoled myself in knowing I could bring this up for many months to come. Instead, I quickly found another pair and opened them, holding them out to Atsede who, at last, met my eyes with a warning glare. I felt a tear trickle down my cheek from the supressed laughter.

Minutes later, Filseta had pushed her son into the world, and was lying on her side, cradling him close. After three girls, I smiled at Filseta's new boy, knowing that's what she was hoping for. Atsede and I offered our congratulations, and, when the placenta was delivered, and her bleeding had stemmed, made our way quietly back through the curtains, leaving Filseta and the baby to rest alone together. I looked at Atsede, who groaned as I opened my mouth, knowing that I would make the most of this opportunity to tease her about what had happened.

Atsede

'No, she didn't!' I was laughing in earnest now, listening to Selam regale me with this morning's story. 'I have to go and see this.'

Making my way through the two doors that closed off the rooms of Delivery from the rest of the hospital, I stepped into the sunshine bathing the red tiles with a warm glow. Looking around me, I saw the wild roses were in bloom now, smiling at the thought of the tangle of dark green leaves and thorns that grew tenaciously over my mother's *sahrbet*, knowing she would step out to the same view. As Selam had promised, the windows of the temporary Neonatal Unit, tucked into a corner of the Surgical Ward that had previously served as an isolation area, were thrown open. The nurses gathered there, their long dresses colourful under their white gowns, with sandalled feet planted easily on the ground and elbows resting on the sandstone mantel, were laughing and teasing. Rahel, slight and dark like many of her Oromia people, with her oval-shaped face and strong chin, had her hair braided differently from normal, long lengths gathered at her crown then trailing down her back. Next to her stood Tsega, the colour of her light eyes as striking as ever, a contrast to her *tikur* colouring, and, slightly older, the matronly Almaz, whose slim figure had filled out with each of her seven children, smiling indulgently through the window.

As I approached them, I called out a greeting, asking after their health, their families', their friends'. The questions bounced back and forth between the four of us until Rahel, grinning, turned to me. 'Have you heard what your *dooriye* Indie panicked about this morning?'

'Selam did mention something about *keywey*...' I started, before a groan from Indie interrupted. Her pale, heart-shaped face appeared in the window, blue eyes, pink cheeks, and yellow hair so different from ours, I thought for the first time in long time, as I saw her in contrast to the nurses.

'Don't any of you have work to do!' Indie's indignant voice only caused more laughter. I smiled though, proud of her growing knowledge of Amharic, and increasing acceptance among the staff as a midwife in her own right, rather than just a guest of Dr

Rita. A few months ago, she would have been mortified at making such a mistake. Now, despite the blush that crept up across her cheeks, I could see she enjoyed the teasing, understanding that these moments of playfulness were what brought us together, and enabled us to keep going through the difficulties.

Laughing, Rahel, Tsega, and Almaz moved aside, allowing me to take their place at the windowsill, before blowing kisses in Indie's direction, receiving narrowed eyes in return, and scattering in different directions, Rahel and Tsega back into the Surgical Ward, and Almaz towards the Medical.

'Indie. *Mah ah roo?* What happened!? You forgot about the butter?' My exclamation was met with a long-suffering sigh.

'*Ere*, actually, Atsede, you are my *astamari*, my teacher, and you never told me! This is all your fault. How was I supposed to know about this?' I couldn't help but smile at her outrage.

'But Sabrina is fine, yes? So, you don't have to worry.' She smiled back, shaking her head slightly, leaning forward to brush her fingers over my hair, twisted alternatively into thick and narrow braids running over the length of my head, gathered underneath themselves at the nape of my neck.

'I like this. Who did it?'

'Hana, she's practising. What do you think?'

'*Konjo*, it's beautiful. It suits you. I still prefer *ibab*, the snakes, though.'

'It isn't *ibab*! But yes, I know you do.' I looked around her, into the Neonatal Unit, the two resuscitaires lined up neatly, awaiting new patients, and the cots beside them both occupied by sleeping babies. Samira was lying on the bright yellow of one of the low campbeds set up next to her baby, catching my eye and nodding a greeting. I turned back to Indie. 'Are you finished here, now, then? No emergency situation after all?'

'Ha. Ha.'

'Shall we go then? You can come and help in Delivery. We've quite a few women today.'

Indie turned to Samira, checking that she wasn't needed. As Samira waved her off, Indie paused to lay a hand gently on a sleeping Sabrina, smiling down at the peaceful little girl and saying something quietly. Edging her way past the cots, Indie appeared a moment later through the swinging doors, and together we walked back up the length of the veranda towards Delivery.

'You know, Indie, if I'm supposed to be teaching you about Gurage culture, I should tell you that you're likely to find *keywey* on the heads of lots of people, not only on newborns.' She looked at me, interested, and gestured for me to continue. 'Children from the villages sometimes have uvulectomies performed by the *Fugah*, except they believe it's a tonsillectomy. *Keywey* is used then as well, placed on the fontanelle in the belief it'll stop the tonsils growing back.' She picked up the slight derision in my voice.

'You don't believe that then, Atse?'

'No, of course not. It's *kaws*, crazy. And dangerous. The blades are rusty, and the *Fugah* don't understand anatomy. Many children die because of it. Not so much anymore, but before, ah, many children.'

'Like circumcision?'

'Yes, exactly.'

Nodding, Indie carried on walking. As soon as we passed through the doors, propped open with a large rock one of the staff had found in the grass outside, I heard my name called. Smiling at Indie, I bade her farewell and made my way to the bedside of a young woman, Genet, who had had her second baby during the night. The baby wasn't sucking properly, she told me, showing her already reddened nipples awkwardly shaped from where they had been pulled into her baby's mouth at the wrong angle. Wincing in sympathy, I settled down next to her, motioning for the baby. Finding a glove in my pocket, I slipped a finger into the baby's mouth, checking for tongue tie. Satisfied that wasn't the reason, I passed the baby back, motioning for Genet to put him to the breast. As soon as she tried, I saw immediately what was making things difficult, and with a few adjustments in his position, moving Genet's hands and arms to better support her baby's head and back, Genet smiled in relief.

'Better?' I asked, not really needing to. 'Remember how you're holding him now, okay? This is perfect. He was too far around, the first time, so he couldn't properly find your nipple. It might still be a bit sore as the redness fades, but you should be able to feel that it's better now?' Genet nodded happily, looking grateful. I sat a moment longer, watching to make sure her baby stayed in position.

'Indie and I are going in with Asnakech and the twins!' Selam's voice called out from the sink used to scrub up before entering the obstetric theatres. I leaned back, looking around the corner towards her. She already had one of the thick plastic aprons wrapped around her, covering her from shoulder to ankle, with feet encased in white clogs far too big for any of the midwives, and a blue paper mask held loosely at her side. Behind her, Indie looked similar.

'*Eshe*, okay.' I called back, relieved at this, then turned to the Delivery boards to put a tick next to her name. Asnakech, who was from our village, had been getting more and more agitated about the pain spanning the width of her body, from hip bone to hip bone. She had been on my mind since arriving an hour ago, and I was sure her scar was starting to dehisce. It seemed Dr Rita thought so too. In the few minutes I had to sit studying the boards, I finalised plans in my mind for each of the women under our care. It would be a busy day; of that I was sure. But then again, almost all our days were busy. Glancing around, I wondered what else needed doing, besides guiding women through their births. There was a stack of notes on the desk, belonging to the women discharged overnight, which needed taking back to the medical record rooms. Next to that, one of the blood pressure cuffs sat forlornly, with seams frayed so badly it was no longer holding the air needed to compress the brachial artery and then slowly allow the blood to flow once more, with a midwife listening for the muffled knocking sounds. There was a scrap of paper resting over, with a scribbled note: 'This tells lies.' I couldn't help but smile, remembering how I had been greeted by a frantic student midwife one afternoon last week, who'd come running to tell me that the woman she was caring for had a blood pressure of 50/20. Despite the initial rush of adrenaline that raced through my veins with her declaration, and after leaping up to look through the connecting windows to the beds of the antenatal room, expecting to see her moribund, collapsed on a bed, with desperate relatives gathering around trying to rouse her, when I caught sight of the woman in question, standing with one hand on her lower back, and the other bent at the elbow leaning against the wall, smiling at the man sitting on the chair next to her, clearly having just come through a contraction and now chatting easily, I smiled.

'Amarech', I had started, trying to disguise my amusement, 'calm down, and take a look at her. Do you really believe that's her blood pressure?'

'But Sister Atsede, I checked twice! It was the same both times.' Her earnest eyes were wide and round, and she was still panting slightly in her fear.

'She's conscious, talking, smiling, standing.'

'Yes.'

'Amarech, a woman with a BP of 50/20 will, I can honestly say, be none of those things. Let me see the BP cuff.' She held it out in front of her, and sure enough, I recognised it. 'Okay, bring the students here.'

Within a few minutes, Amarech and her classmates, eight of them altogether, had gathered in the small space that made up the midwives' area, some sitting on the desk or sharing a chair, some standing. I asked Amarech to take us through her findings, smiling with reassurance, then asked them all to stand up and look at the woman whose BP was causing such a stir. Another contraction having passed, she was now standing easily at the side of her bedspace, retying the *shajsh* that bound her hair and reaching for the bottle of Mirinda balanced on the windowsill.

'What Amarech discovered today, and what all of you will at some time during your life as a midwife, is this: as good as technology and equipment is, the midwife is better. You cannot just unthinkingly rely on the results of the investigations you do, whether that's a blood pressure or an ultrasound. You have to remember to see at the whole picture. Don't look at the numbers, look at the woman.' I saw Amarech blush, and remembered my own discomfiture when something similar had happened to me during my days as a student. 'But what Amarech did was exactly right. She was concerned about a finding, checked it twice to make sure it wasn't a mistake, and sought help from a senior midwife. Much better than what I did in a similar situation.' I watched Amarech relax, and saw that I'd piqued the interest of the girls, sighing because that meant that one of them, surely, would ask…

'What situation, Sister Atsede?'

As expected. 'I was a first year, and for the first time was about to catheterise a real woman. So I got everything ready, put my gloves on, placed the catheter, got fluid flowing into the bag, pushed in saline to inflate the balloon, and wrote it all down, a little surprised at how easy it had been, how little soreness the woman had felt, and how simple finding the urethra had been, and relieved as anything that it had gone so smoothly. I was so busy making sure I cleaned up everything, that I didn't check with her to see how it felt. A few minutes later, when my mentor, who was terrifying by the way, was supporting the woman into theatre and shrieked, I went running. The woman, believing she had a catheter, had felt the urge to urinate, and had done so. Only to find it running down her legs, on to the floor, and into the shoes of my mentor. It turns out I hadn't catheterised her urethra, but her cervix, and the fluid I'd seen was amniotic, from where, somehow, I'd pushed the catheter up and into the sac.' Laughter from my audience. 'If I hadn't been so focused on the steps of catheterisation, and ticking the boxes in my mind, and had just instead engaged with the woman while I was catheterising her, I'm sure I would have realised.' Shaking my head, I continued. 'So, it just goes to show. Remember, you are midwives, caring for women. Not technicians, reporting numbers. Okay, off you go, get back to your cases.'

With a clattering of chairs being scraped back, the students had scattered across the wards, and I'd turned back to my work, eyes flicking between boards and beds. I leant towards the theatres, catching sight of Indie going back in quickly, leaving Selam and the resuscitaire with the two small babies whose lusty cries were now filling the room. Wondering in passing why she'd gone back in, but distracted by the wheelchair being pushed around the corner to the Delivery Room, I stood to meet whoever it belonged to. A heartbeat later, the sweet, oval-shaped face of Maregnesh, a friend of mine, and just about everyone's, from the village, appeared smiling shyly. As well as being my friend, Maregnesh and I were also related through *gowza*, through our tribes, as we were both *Yederaratib Ergah*, making us as close as sisters.

'Maregu! Is it time? Is this little girl finally ready to meet me?' I'd seen Maregnesh all through her pregnancy, but hadn't realised it was time. Her smile grew as she nodded. 'Come on in then, find a bed and lie down, let me have a look at you.'

She heaved herself out of the wheelchair before making her way between the plaid curtains and trying to find a comfortable way to sit on the waiting bed, rearranging her long dress so that it could be easily lifted above her bump. After checking her blood pressure, pulse, and temperature, I watched as Maregnesh lay down. Something prickled at the edge of my mind. I couldn't identify what exactly, but something was wrong here. Whether it was the way she moved, or the way she held herself, I wasn't sure. It didn't seem to be anything specific, and I wasn't sure how to explain it. But intuition is simply reality being processed too fast for the conscious mind to comprehend, and mine was on edge. 'Maregu, have you been having pains? Have your waters gone?'

'Not pains, I don't think, but my back hurts, and it's been very sensitive here.' As she said it she touched the side of her bump, low down on the left, and winced. It was unusual to have a localised specific pain in the abdomen itself. Around the flanks or back, yes, but not in the place Maregnesh had indicated. Even having spent only minutes with Maregnesh, I felt on edge.

'Give me a moment.' Laying a reassuring hand on her arm, I turned away from Maregnesh and stepped through the curtains. 'Indie?'

'Mmm?' Her chin rested on one hand, the other holding a pen that moved quickly across the paper as she filled in the details on Asnakech's notes. It stilled as she half-turned towards, watching me approach.

'There is something happening.'

'Okay. What's going on? What do you need?

'I don't know.'

She paused at that, took her head off her hand and shifted in her chair to face me, tilting her head to the side.

'Okay. What do you want me to do?'

Her confidence in my judgement steadied my rapid heartbeat. But I didn't know what to do, or what I wanted Indie to do. I looked back to Maregnesh, lying on her side. My hand still held the pinard I had placed against her stomach. It had felt normal, and when I listened, her baby's heartbeat had also sounded normal. But her eyes were different, glazed slightly, and a there was a waver to her voice. Her pulse was normal and her blood pressure. On paper, there was no real reason to suspect anything was wrong. And yet.

'Shall I ask Dr Rita to come and assess?'

I nodded, watching Maregnesh closely. Indie stood up and walked out. I alternated between my seat at Maregnesh's side, and the windows that lined the room, letting in light and fresh air, unable to settle while we waited. I'm not sure what Indie told Dr Rita, but it felt like only minutes later that I watched as they rounded the corner and walked down the length of the low sandstone building that housed the operating theatres and the Delivery Room. Indie was talking animatedly, and gesticulating, while Dr Rita listened. I turned to Maregnesh, smiling.

'I've asked the doctor to come and see you. Your baby is peaceful right now, and everything I have checked has been normal. But I know you feel strange, and looking at you, you don't seem yourself, your face has changed. So, let's just see what Dr Rita says.'

The swish of a door followed a few moments later. Dr Rita nodded a greeting, holding out a hand for the notes, and introducing herself to Maregnesh. Behind her, Indie caught my eye then inclined her head to the desk. I nodded, and she slipped around Dr Rita before sitting at the desk and picking up the pen again. Taking a deep breath, I turned to explain why I had asked her to come. Dr Rita listened intently, and I was grateful for this, then sat to read quickly through Maregnesh's notes. She turned over the last page, eyes skimming the ultrasound performed a month ago, before closing the notes, and reaching to lay a hand on Maregnesh's chest, feeling, I knew, for her temperature, her heart rate, the clamminess of her skin. Moments later, she leaned back against the chair, and looked up at me.

'So, Atsede, what do you want to do now?'

I'd been thinking about this since I'd first looked at Maregnesh. 'I think she should have an ultrasound, first.'

'Then that is what we will do.' Dr Rita's reply came, as she tipped her head to one side thoughtfully. 'I'll bring it here.'

'Thank you.' Relief washed over me as Dr Rita stood. I smiled at Maregnesh. 'Maregu, do you understand what we've been saying? Dr Rita is going to give you an ultrasound, then we can have a look at your baby and see what's happening.'

The next 10 minutes passed in a single moment. In one breath, Dr Rita handed me the gel to spread across Maregnesh's stomach while she turned on the machine, and in the next I heard her exclamation of surprise as the almost complete abruption of Maregnesh's placenta flashed across the screen in front us. In the next I was tying her surgical gown on as the anaesthetist administered the general anaesthetic. With every second mattering, Dr Rita had asked Indie to scrub in as the assistant, to hand over instruments, hold onto clamps, staunch the flow of blood with white packs. As Dr Rita cut through the muscles of Maregnesh's uterus, a wave of blood spilled out of her. Dr Rita reached in to find the head of her baby, shaking her head in utter disbelief as she lifted him out, Maregnesh's first child, crying, moving, alive. I reached out to take him, unable to comprehend what I was seeing, overwhelmed in that moment that the baby had survived, and in the moments after she came around from the anaesthesia that Maregnesh had as well.

It was a momentous achievement, discharging Maregnesh and her baby, both healthy, a week later. She had needed blood, donated of course by Indie, and had felt weak and unsteady for days. But I go cold every time I think of that day, and how different it could have been. It was also a memory to hold on to, as just a few days after I walked next to Maregnesh as she was pushed in a wheelchair to the waiting *bajaj* that would take her home, I would be walking next to the body of a woman carried on a litter who hadn't been so fortunate.

It had started like many mornings; busy but not unusually so. At last, a few minutes of fresh air and bright sunshine. Sitting on the low brick wall, back against the cool sandstone of the operating theatres, I closed my eyes, turning my head to the brightness, and enjoyed the warmth seeping into my skin. For just a few seconds I was a young girl again, lying next to my sisters with arms outstretched in the long grass of the savannah, faces to the sun, listening to the chattering of insects and birds and monkeys, the pile of firewood we had been collecting heaped at our sides. Suddenly, the slamming of a door broke my reverie, and blinking I turned towards the source.

I watched as Indie came swiftly out of the surgical ward, walking with a single-minded purpose that I knew meant her patient wasn't going to make it. It would be difficult for her, losing a woman whose veins now carried her blood. This time of year was always busy, and I was grateful that she was now capable of managing the intensive cases. It freed me up to carry on with keeping everything else going. But I knew another woman dying would weigh down her usually light heart. I had felt that way too, all those years ago when I was first charged with caring for critically ill patients. I still do, but it is tempered by an acceptance that life is tinged with devastation as well as celebration. Nowhere is that more apparent than in the birth room. The fragile mortality of life is challenged here every day. Indie said she is envious of my Catholic faith, and how it has helped me to understand that there are things way beyond my control that I can't change, but that I can believe will happen for a reason. I'm not sure if she's right, but there is a comfort in knowing that life, however and whenever it comes to an end, did have meaning and did matter, not just to those who loved and who were loved in return, but as part of a bigger idea. It doesn't stop the pain of loss, but there is a peace and a beauty and a comfort in knowing that where they have gone, they are not alone, that the end here is the beginning there, and that a great presence, quietly but eternally, is in the background.

We had talked just days ago about faith and hope and grief, sitting at the side of Indie's neonatal patients, several of whom were unlikely to pull through. And in the end, we realised that these feelings are all just manifestations of love. Hope is for love to come, grief is for love left behind, faith is a belief in love. When I first became a midwife, I was told to care *for* my patients, but not to care *about* them. It seems a fine distinction, but it is there nonetheless. I understand why we were taught this, but I disagree now as fervently as I disagreed then. Midwifery is the expression of the vast spectrum of human experience laid bare, captured in a few moments, and as we walk the gamut with women, we owe it to them, and to ourselves, to understand this. We have to love. When things go well, and when things don't. As I watched Indie plead with Dr Rita for a deliverance from fate for her patient, I saw with a sudden clarity what love meant in reality, the toll it takes, the struggle. Like me, she was a midwife who cares about, not just for, and now she would have to face the consequences of that, and the heartbreak of loss.

There was a moment of quiet on the ward, with just the gentle murmur of women comforting their babies, and the occasional sighing groan of a woman just starting her labour. I wasn't needed there, so I caught Dr Rita's attention, and raised an eyebrow in question. The slightest nod of her head, and I stood, walking over to join them. As I came closer, I could hear the desperation in Indie's voice and she begged for an answer.

'She's dying, Indie.' I reached out to touch her and she turned, taking a moment to register my words. It was as if a veil had been lifted, and I watched her physically respond to the realisation. Her shoulders dropped, her hands stilled and fell to her side. I could see she didn't trust herself to speak, for fear her control would break. Too many times over the last decade I had been here, seen this. These women are my sisters, my aunts, my friends, and still we die in childbirth. Indie hadn't come to terms with that yet, she was fighting. Watching her react, I wondered if she was right. Perhaps I shouldn't have adjusted to death being part of birth. Perhaps fighting is better. But in this instance, the fight wasn't to save Meske's life, it was to let her die in peace.

'Even though this is tragic, Indie, this is not your tragedy. Her family will remember that you cared, that we all cared. So, you can be sad, and shed tears, but remember, however hard this is for you, this is a thousand times harder for her family. And your job isn't finished, yet.'

It felt as though in that single moment, their lives were changed forever. Except, I thought as I sat and watched her daughters fall apart, helpless, it wasn't a single moment, it was a kaleidoscope of moments, all leading to this point in time. The vulnerability of life was breathtaking, especially in the birthing room, where women come so close to oblivion. The thing about courage, though, is that just a little is enough to make all the difference in the world. And Meske's mother was full of courage, sitting silently with her daughter through it all. While there would be no chance for the wounds on her daughter's body to heal and then fade, the scars of her experience would be there, carried instead by her mother, her husband, her sisters, her children. And her midwives, I thought sadly, sometime later, after it was over and Meske had begun her final journey home, watching Indie's retreating back. I knew where she was going, to the Neonatal Unit, to Sabrina, her miracle patient. It was what she needed now, I thought, to see evidence of the tenacity of life in the face of the cruelty of death. It was that same need that would carry her back to the Delivery Room that evening, that would keep her at the bedside of the women who came through our doors, placing her hands on their *den,* feeling for the movements of their unborn babies, listening to the sounds of coming life.

Hours later, I heard Indie's voice call out. I had meant to make sure she was okay before now, but a woman with severe pre-eclampsia needing close management had kept me away. With my patient now trying to rest through the initial stages of an induced labour, I had sought out a beloved cousin, Betsalot, who had given birth to her third baby, a daughter she named Beza, in the night. We were drinking *kawa* and eating *kollo,* talking quietly in the cool, dim lighting of the postnatal room, the sister of Betsalot's husband telling us about the scene unfolding in the Emergency Room as she passed by. What exactly it was, she wasn't sure, but there was now a donkey tied up there. I was laughing at that as Indie's disembodied voice came once more. She sounded steady though, I thought, and as she rounded the corner in search of me, her whole body seemed calmer. Gone was the tightly wound distress that had held her rigid earlier today; instead she was relaxed, moving easily.

'Atse, there you are. Betsalot, *en kuan des alesh,* your baby is beautiful!' she said, leaning over to move the corner of the woven *gabi* so she could see. 'Oh', she whispered, '*Miski,* such a sweet girl!' Betsalot looked at her daughter proudly, tracing the tip of a finger over the arch of her eyebrow, before reaching over to kiss Indie on the cheek in greeting. 'Betsalot, I'm really sorry to interrupt, but can I have Atse please?'

She waved me away, and I held out a hand for Indie to help me up. As we walked back around the corner, I held her back for a moment.

'Are you okay, Indie?' She turned to me, and nodded, smiling reassuringly. 'Really?'

'Yes, Atsde , *dehenenegn*, I am okay. Thank you.'

'Okay. So, what do you need me for?'

Indie shook her head in bewilderment, 'I don't know. But Selam wants me to go with her somewhere, and she is very insistent. Will you look after Filseta please? She's inside.'

'Of course,' I replied, wondering what Selam was up to. 'Tell me about your woman?'

'Thank you. Filseta, yes. So, fourth baby, three previous straightforward pregnancies and births, no complications this time. I just examined her, she was eight centimeters, very soft and stretchy, with bulging membranes. Blood pressure and pulse perfect, baby's heart perfect. I was counting her contractions one more time, but I think as soon as she stands up, and baby's head comes down, those membranes will go and she'll deliver. I've written all the notes, and prepared the instruments. She knows you're coming. I'd like to be back before that baby comes along, but I think it could be very soon!'

'Got it, thank you. I'll keep an eye on her. Her name is Filseta, yes?' Indie nodded, hanging up her gown on the pegs just inside the midwives' area, and made her way out of the door. Tipping up the small china *sini* in my hand to finish the last of the *kawa* within, I felt the gritty beans that hadn't been fully ground catch on my tongue, and moved them to crunch between my teeth, then took the *sini* to the sink, swishing water around the inside. Leaving it upside down to dry, balanced on a towel on top of the autoclave, I searched for my phone on top of the fridge next to it, where it had been for the last few hours. In the villages, electricity is unreliable, often disappearing for days at a time, so the extension cord on top of the fridge nearly always plays host to a tangle of cables charging an array of phones, torches, radios, and once even an electric toothbrush, which caused much amusement as it started vibrating violently in the early hours. Seeing it hidden under a torch, I checked the time, pleased to see it wasn't too late. Turning back to the desk, I moved handfuls of notes stapled in the folded blue card that held them together, wanting to know Filseta's history. As promised, they were sitting neatly to one side, opened on the page containing Indie's small, precise writing. I glanced over them, then flicked through the previous deliveries. Three girls, I realised, wondering what her fourth would be. Tucked against the tray containing the notes of the high-risk women, those with pre-eclampsia, placenta praevia, a high number of pregnancies, PPROM, was the pinard I needed. Taking it up, I stepped over the small wooden *burchama*, stool, tucked in next to the desk, and made my way to the only bed with the curtains pulled around.

Inside, Filseta was squatting by the footstep, hands clasped around the metal bedposts, one on top of each other, nails white with the tightness of her grip. Waiting until the contraction finished, I busied myself rearranging the white material thrown over the examination couch, smoothing wrinkles and ensuring the worst of the worn rubber was covered. Used until they fell apart, the strips of material provided a clean surface for the women to sit or lie on, and soaked up some of the fluids of birth. As Filseta's groaning eased, she looked up, nodding a greeting in my direction. I wondered if I recognised her. Something in the roundness of her eyes and her high cheekbones felt familiar, but I couldn't quite place her.

'Filseta, I think Indie told you that I would be here to look after you until she came back? I'm Atsede, the senior midwife.'

'Atsede, of course. You're Kidane's daughter?' She smiled at me kindly. 'I knew your father well. He always bought *fehke besehr*, goat meat, from me for you girls for *Giyorgis kara*, St George's Day.' Her sentence was punctuated by heavy breaths as she recovered from the contraction.

I smiled, now able to place her, hair bound in a colourful *shajsh*, a thick stick raised to shoulder level ready to bring down on the rump of an errant goat. *Yuiskiss, yuiskiss!* she would call to them, followed by the thwack of wood on bony hide as she guided her flock along the well-trodden paths worn between the *gwaro*. All the patron saints have their own day here. Filseta had remembered well, my father's favourite saint had always been Giyorgis, so on the twenty-third day of each month we would prepare *kawa*, scramble eggs, and cook a thick, spicy *wot* made with the meat my father bought. Half a kilo, for 10 of us. It seemed so extravagant, but my father insisted. It was a fact that, years later, delighted Indie when I told her.

'But St George is English!' she had said, eyes alight with laughter. 'Your father was a very wise man indeed!' She had taken up his tradition with great enthusiasm, bringing bottles of lukewarm Fanta Pineapple and baskets of popcorn for the staff at the Clinic every month on the twenty-third. After little Raphael was born, on the thirteenth day of the month, the day dedicated to the archangel who shares his name, she realised she was now responsible for both. Giyorgis for her country, Raphael for her son.

I smiled at Filseta, who had stood up from her squat and was now rocking from side to side, hands on the bed, head on her shoulder. Judging by the way she moved, the way she sounded, I could see why Indie had prepared everything for the birth. I didn't think it would be long either. I wondered in passing where Selam had taken Indie, then remembered what Asnakech's sister had being saying about the donkey, and wondered briefly if they were connected. As Filseta began to groan once again, I forgot about it altogether, instead concentrating on the woman in front of me. The minutes passed, and Filseta stood and squatted in turn, her groaning turning to the whooping *oooeeewii, oooeeeewii* that women often make to help them handle the intense pressure of their baby's head moving down. It faded with the contraction, and Filseta wiped a hand across her face, looking in surprise at the sweat gathered in the creases of her palm.

'Filseta, your baby will come soon. Do you want to stay like this? Or move onto the bed? Which is best for you?' She regarded me blankly for a moment, trying to work out what I was saying. It was a look I recognised, one often seen in the eyes of women on the brink of birth, in the space between consciousness and oblivion. If I could help it, I didn't usually speak to women at this time, but the floors of the Delivery Room weren't as clean as the bed, and I would need to bring more cloths to put down.

Her mind now having understood what I had asked, Filseta motioned to the bed. Moving alongside her, one hand on her back, the other under her elbow, I helped her up. She lay for a few moments on her side, before rearing up on to her hands and knees with the coming contraction. As she did so, her dress caught up and I saw the first glimpse of her baby's head. Shaking my own ruefully at myself for not anticipating that the change in position and the movement of her pelvis as she climbed onto the bed would advance the birth, I quickly pulled on a glove and reached out. As the contraction peaked, the baby's head came down further. I wriggled my fingers uncomfortably, having, in my haste, managed to get two fingers into the same hole, and tried, unsuccessfully, to slip my other hand into the remaining glove. I didn't want to move my hands, certain that with the next contraction the baby would come, so I stood, feeling ridiculous, one hand cramped uncomfortably inside a glove, the other wiggling uselessly trying to get the other some way on. It was at that exact moment that the curtain moved slightly. I looked up to see who it was, and heard Indie's quiet whisper.

'Atse, Filse, I came back. Can I come through?'

My initial feelings of relief were quickly replaced with dread. I would never hear the end of this if Indie caught me as I was. Too late, I realised, as Filsete groaned her consent, and Indie slipped through. She took in the scene in front of her, and I could see the control it took to keep her laughter from spilling out and disturbing Filseta's calm. Her shoulders shaking, and tears in her eyes, one hand went to her mouth as she tried to catch my eye. Keeping my own gaze stubbornly on Filseta, I felt rather than saw Indie leave. A handful of seconds later she was back, a fresh pack of gloves opened and held in front of her. She offered them to me, still silently trembling with mirth, and I grudgingly took them, peeling off the previous ones and slipping them on in one movement, hands back beneath Filseta as the final contraction came, and her baby's body followed his head out and into my hands. I looked at the cord tethering him to the placenta, and widened my eyes in interest. Three true knots. He must have been moving all over her uterus as he grew to tangle himself up like that, I thought, also unlooping it from around his neck and across his shoulder.

'Not a single word,' I growled quietly to Indie as I passed Filseta, who had moved onto her side, her new son, pulling the blanket she'd been using as a pillow out from underneath her head and placing it gently over them.

Fresh tears escaping her eyes, Indie shook her head. 'Even if I wanted to, there's too many things to choose from, I couldn't settle on just one.'

I threw her what I hoped was a withering look before turning back to Filseta. '*Enkuan des alesh*, Filseta. A boy!'

'Big, too,' Indie added, looking at the chunky arm that reached just outside the blanket. '*Enkuan des alesh*, Filse.'

She smiled at both of us in turn, before closing her eyes and leaning back. In her arms, her son moved against her, searching for the nipple. Without opening her eyes, Filseta reach up to guide him, and the grimace that passed briefly over her face told us he had found it, latching on with the force of a newborn. After Filseta's placenta had delivered, and with the mother and her new baby tucked in together resting, I led Indie back through the curtains, sighing at the inevitable torrent of teasing that was about to come my way.

'Okay, Indie, let's hear it.' I tried, and failed, to hide my smile as Indie looked at me, grinning.

'Well, Atsede…'

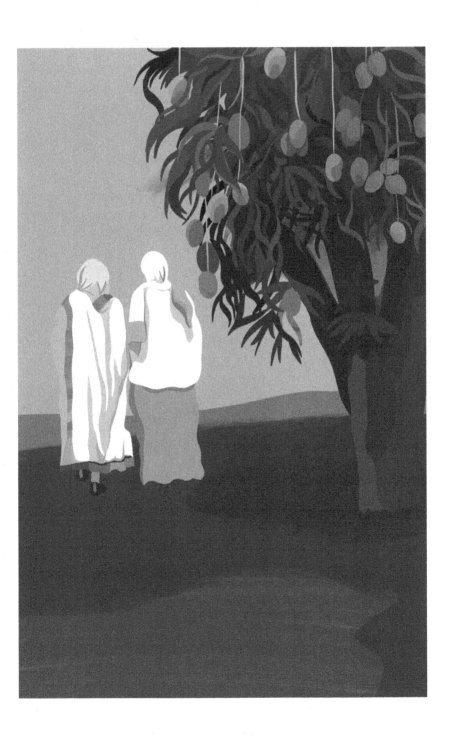

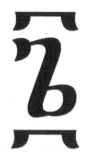

6

Meseret

Indie

I had never witnessed such a visceral reaction to loss. Her whole being screamed with grief; her movements subdued, her voice deadened. It was as if her spirit had left her, as well as her son. Seeing it was all the more shocking in how it stood in stark contrast with the usual stoicism of the Gurage women in the face of catastrophe. I looked to Atsede, unsure how to respond, but her eyes were focused on the woman on the floor in front of us. She crouched down next to her, reaching out. 'Ah, Birtukan. I'm so sorry.'

With that, tears leaked from Birtukan's eyes. 'I don't understand. This is witchcraft. This is bad, dark magic. Why would he do it?' Drained and exhausted, she collapsed back on to the mat on the floor, staring with blank eyes at the wall in front of her. Shaking her head, Atsede stood and motioned me to join her on the *borchama* stools spaced along the length of the room. We had come for the *luxor*. Birtukan's son had been found the evening before. I hadn't known him well, but his family *gwaro* ran the length of Atsede's, and Birtukan had always shown great kindness to Atsede and, since I first stepped under the arch of palm leaves into Atsede's family four years ago, to me too.

'What will happen to Birtukan?' I asked Atsede as we traced our way through the long grass. Reaching out either side, I drew the strands through my hands, collecting seeds before throwing handfuls back into the grass. Atsede had told me they always did this as children, after their grandmother told them she wanted their meadows to be the thickest of all, and the only way to do that was to make sure the birds didn't take the seeds and fly off with them.

'The village will stay with her and, in time, she will heal. The fire inside of her burns brighter than the fire around her. It's difficult though. Broken-hearted people no longer look after themselves. They are too full of grief to see past their trauma. The *wog* says they are between worlds, which is why we have to take care of them, to show them there's reason to stay in this one.' Atsede, too, was collecting seeds. I watched as she threw a handful, the wind catching the lighter ones, cascading them out over the path, and thought about her answer. I'd heard her talk about the *wog* before, but there had always been something else to do or someone else to see to before I'd had a chance to ask about what, or who, exactly it is. This was my chance though, and as we rounded the gully carved through the hillside and entered the dappled shade of the forest, I stopped, wondering if I should ask, or if Atsede was too lost in thought to be distracted by my question. But as she turned, she smiled, and there was the familiar look of mixed exasperation and amusement on her face. I grinned back, and asked.

'Atse, who is this *wog*?'

I loved hearing Atsede talking about the Gurage ways. Her voice changed and it thickened with pride and happiness. And while she scolded me for asking too much, too often, telling me I was worse than a little child, I knew she enjoyed it really. I could see she was thinking about how to answer my question. I'd heard her, and others, talk about the *wog* before, always with respect in their voices, often bordering on reverence, so had some idea of who I thought he was. Atsede confirmed it, explaining he was the guardian of Gurage ways, able to offer suggestions to resolve disputes, or mitigate curses, within the framework of Gurage beliefs. An unenviable task, I thought to myself, given the conflicting influences on so many of the Gurage: religion, modernity, familial ties. But then again, being Gurage seems to sit at the forefront of their identity, jostling for that position only with their faith. Certainly I've seen that in Atsede, her friends and their families, and I'm sure their ties to each other through the complex *gowza* system explain the peace that exists between Orthodox, Catholic, and Muslim Gurages. I've never known religion to be a reason for dissent, and when I asked Atsede about it my suspicions were confirmed. Whether they follow the Bible or the Qur'an, the bonds of the *gowza* unite them all. At the end of Ramadan, our neighbours bring us bowls of rich oat soup, and during the week-long celebrations of Meskel, the Finding of the True Cross, we cook lentil *wot* to be shared by all. At weddings or funerals, two feasts are prepared, one using halal meat bought from the Muslim butchers, the other for Christians. Two parallel lines form, snaking back from the different tables, arranged opposite each other, upon which the dishes, identical in taste and presentation, are served from big, shallow, black clay *bitr*. It's symbolic of the approach of the Gurages to peaceful coexistence; while they use different meat, the dish is the same.

We picked our way carefully down the steep gully, holding on to the slim trunks of the towering eucalyptus. During the rains it was almost impassable, not that that stopped Atsede from visiting her family, with me and the boys in tow. With sandals in our hands, and long dresses tied up above our knees, we would go slowly, trying to jump from hillock to rock, but often giving up and simply accepting that the rich red mud would end up coating everything. Those walks through the gully were a favourite with the boys, who relished the chance to splash through puddles and squish their toes in the earth. By the end of it, they were indistinguishable from one another, Raphael's light hair and Mesmora's dark skin both coloured the red-brown of the soil. Several buckets of rainwater sloshed over them went some way in cleaning it off, but given that they would spend the day playing outside anyway, it seemed pointless to insist. The real bath would come later that evening, back in our house in the town, when we would light big fires and warm up the water, hand them bars of soap, and keep a wary distance as they splashed and blew bubbles. Only Yordannos was brave enough to venture close, ensuring the soap found all the creases and crevices it needed to.

Thankfully, it was dry now, the ground sandy. Reaching the bottom, I turned to hold a hand up to Atsede, helping her down the last incline. Despite her insistence that she was as agile as the *gimbe*, the antelope, that leapt across the grasslands in the dawn, her growing bump made balancing more difficult, and she took it gratefully. As we reached the dirt track leading back to the road, Atsede sighed with relief to see a *bajaj* waiting, and settled into the seat at the back, one hand going to her head.

'I haven't drunk enough today,' she said regretfully, 'and I knew that *kawa* would give me a headache.'

'*Nikit*, Atse.' I felt for her, and had wanted her to stay behind while

I represented us both at the *luxor*. She wouldn't hear of it though, insisting on coming too, despite the long walk under the hot sun. '*Aye zohr.*' They were two of my favourite phrases in Guraginya, neither with an equivalent in English, but both used often here, indicating affection and empathy, expressing with just those words that if the speaker could take any sadness or discomfort from the one the words are directed at, they would do so in a heartbeat.

Atsede smiled, before resting her head to the side against the roughly painted window. She laughed suddenly, pointing to a familiar sticker, peeling slightly, on the window, where the logo and name of our Clinic were stamped, along with our numbers and the assurance we would be there all hours of the day and night. I chatted inconsequentially with the driver as we made our way back along the length of asphalt road that ran through the town, before turning off to the left, dodging zebu and goats browsing the rough grass that grew across the track to the Clinic.

'I didn't tell you', Atsede spoke up as the *bajaj* careened around a huddle of fattail sheep, 'Dawit said there was a *gwencha*, a hyena, on the road this morning! Must have been one of the trucks from the quarry. A *bajaj* wouldn't kill a hyena. I wonder who got the eyebrows.'

'The eyebrows?'

'Absolutely, the eyebrows. They're good luck. If you have a hyena's eyebrow, then you will be rich. There would have been a tussle over those this morning, I tell you.'

'In my country, it's a rabbit's foot.'

We smiled at each other, enjoying finding threads of connection between our experiences and upbringings. There were many times that not only were our ways of behaving different, but our ways of thinking, and yet, more often than we had imagined, for each of these moments there were many more when we found things to bring us together, rather than set us apart.

The rest of the day passed quickly, with patients in the Emergency Room keeping Atsede in its cool depths as I took the opportunity the lull in antenatal appointments provided to catch up on tasks we put aside when busy. The instruments used for suturing wounds, removing contraceptive implants, and changing dressings, needed sterilising. Wrapped in small squares of white cloth cut from a sheet brought from England, they were placed in the autoclave, balanced on three big rocks spaced around the fire lit underneath. Watching as the needle spun in the dial as the water within the metal drum turned to steam, it needed constant attendance to ensure the flames stayed hot enough to keep the pressure up. Gauze needed preparing, cut from a long roll and folded in on itself into small squares, then packed away in metal tins, ready to be sterilised. With the number of patients we were seeing daily steadily increasing, the blue card folders used to hold medical notes needed numbering and stamping. In the late afternoon, with Aster taking over in the Emergency Room, I heard Alem call out to me. Stepping outside, I saw her, mop in hand, gesturing to the flowerbed outside the staff room. Clicking my tongue and hands raised, I circled behind the black and white goats who regularly broke in to the compound to find the succulent leaves of the lower branches of our small avocado tree. They bleated defiantly, hesitant to give up the prize, but eventually relented as I got close enough to give them a sharp slap. Laughing, Alem watched as they scattered, scrambling over the low wall that demarcated the garden area and out of the gates. I turned back to the staff room and peered through the window, smiling as I saw Atsede on a mat on the staffroom floor, fast asleep. Tucked up next to her were Mesmora and Raphael, who must have come in when the sun got too hot. I couldn't help but smile at the three of them, blissfully unaware, pleased that Atsede was resting. Sleeping, I could see the bellies of the boys still rounded out, replete from the glistening watermelon from the mountain slopes, where the rains grew them and the sunshine sweetened them. Atsede had called them 'fluid fruit' once, when the English word for *habhab* proved elusive, and we'd called them that ever since. The tiny sunbirds that nested in the uppermost branches of the swaying Clinic trees were brave enough now to flit in and out of the rooms at will, and their beady eyes had seen the black seeds and dark green rinds lying in small pools of watermelon juice. Calling out to each other, they were swooping down, flashes of bright red and royal blue, picking at them, pausing sometimes to scoop up the sweet, sticky puddles before retreating into the trees.

As the sun sank out of view on the horizon, and the blue skies overhead darkened with coming night, there was a familiar knock at the gates as two young women ducked through. Aster and I had been pulling shutters and doors closed against the mountain cold while Atsede corralled the boys together, making sure shoes were on the right feet and stones had been emptied from pockets. Yordannos was packing her homework away, having spent the last hour at my desk copying out phrases in English, coming to check after each one that she'd got it right. We all looked around, smiling in greeting, and it was clear the taller of the two was in labour. She had her arm slung over the shoulder of the other, and one hand holding the bottom of her bump.

'*Lidgewoj*, boys, *nah*, come.' Mesmora and Raphael approached Atsede, sitting on the bench under the bottlebrush, as she held out a hand to each of them. 'Listen, Yordannos and Aster are going to take you home, okay? We are just going to help this woman and then we will come too.'

They looked around at the newcomers, eyes wide.

'*Ophew*? Sick?' Raphael asked, pointing at them. Atsede smiled and pulled him closer, scooping him on to the bench next to her where she could reach the shoelace that had come undone.

'She's not sick, but she has a tiny baby inside that might come out soon. So mama and me have to help her.' Raphael still looked concerned, but Mesmora nodded sagely, with the air of a child who understood everything there was to understand, before taking his hand, and pulling him out of the gates, Yordannos running after them. Aster waved farewell too, and followed their retreating backs.

'Meseret,' Atsede said, standing to greet her. 'It's started?' The tall woman nodded, looking apprehensive but resolute. I remembered meeting her months ago, listening as she spoke of the pain and trauma of her previous birth, when she'd begged the midwives to stop as they cut her then forced the metal cap of an obstetric vacuum onto her baby's head, pulling without a contraction, one midwife leaning all her weight on Meseret's fundus to force the baby down. In the wrong position, and forced further into it with the damaging fundal pressure, the baby had been unable to move through, so the vacuum had failed, and tears flowing, she had been taken for a caesarean. When her baby was at last handed to her, he looked as battered and bruised as she felt. Now, years later, she was afraid. Atsede and I had spoken to her at length, reassuring her that we did things differently here. The fear in her eyes had started to fade as we said, again and again, that no one here would ever make her do anything she didn't agree to, and she had said she wanted to birth at the Clinic.

True to the agreement we had reached, I showed Meseret and her sister to the birthing room, reassuring them both that this was her space, and she could decide who to bring into it and when. I went on to gently explain that I'd like to do an initial assessment, to check everything was okay, and to give us some idea of how the night might go. Another contraction came and went before she decided, but as the vice-like grip of her uterine muscles loosened, she nodded in consent. As unobtrusively and quickly as I could, I checked her and the baby, happy to find that she was already in advanced labour, and that her baby was coping with it well. I smiled at them both, saying just that, then taking Meseret's sister to the door, showing her the fire Atsede had built just inside the gate, and the two chairs she had pulled around it.

'That is where we will be, *ishi*? Meseret knows that, sometimes, I would like to come and listen to her baby. But I will knock, and wait here until she agrees I can come in. If she feels like the birth is coming, or if she is worried about anything, just call for us, and we will come. *Ishi*?' Meseret's sister nodded in understanding, reaching out to touch my hand in a gesture of gratitude. I smiled. '*Hulum selam new*, everything is at peace, now. We will be at the fire.'

Atsede and I passed the hours quietly, conversation punctuated by easy silence as we watched the sparks dance in the sky. As the tenor of Meseret's groans changed, I found myself waiting at the door more and more often, expecting at any moment to be called in. It wasn't until sometime later that that happened, after I had ventured just beyond the gate to pull some wood from Desu's secret stash inside the wooden hut half built on the neighbouring land. Atsede looked tired, the fire throwing the slightly bruised-looking skin under her eyes into sharp relief, and I worried about her. She should be resting. When I voiced this, though, she had laughed dismissively, claiming that it was far more peaceful here, under the stars next to the flames, than it would be at home, where the boys would use her as a prop in their games, then Dawit would want her to sit with him as he ate. Here, at last, she could sit in solitude, a blanket over her shoulders, feet propped up on the still warm autoclave.

Meseret's sister's slim fingers appeared around the side of the door, pushing it slightly open, before her face peered around.

'She'd like you to come in, now.'

We smiled in acknowledgement, and made our way across the cobbles and up on to the veranda. It was warm and dark inside the room, with just a small, flexible lamp turned on in the corner. Meseret's bag sat on the chair, and her dress was draped over the back of it. It took us a moment to find her, sitting on the blue birth ball, balancing against the bed. I smiled to myself, glancing quickly at Atse. *Told you so,* I mouthed. As we watched, Meseret rose to her feet, the skin of her long legs glistening with sweat. I heard Atsede and Ehuty, Meseret's sister, teasing each other quietly as I made my way to Meseret's side. Not wanting to startle her, I reached out gently, laying a hand on the *gabi* she had pulled over her shoulders.

'Mese, how are you? Are you feeling different now?' She nodded, motioning to her back, her abdomen.

'Pressure, I feel so much pressure. And I have so much *shint*, urine.' She spoke so quietly I could barely catch her words.

'*Ishi.* We have a *popo*, a bedpan, here, so you don't have to go outside. I'll help you.'

Meseret had been right. It was a full bedpan I carried to the toilets a few minutes later. With her bladder empty and out of the way, I hoped her baby would continue to move further down. More contractions came and went as Meseret's groans became deeper, less controlled. Standing at the bedside, she stood on her tiptoes as it came once more. Kneeling just behind her, I could just see the dark hair on the top of her baby's head. With her sister whispering encouragement, Meseret bore down, and as she did so, her baby's head was born, causing her to cry out. My hands were there, waiting, while she panted, hands clenching convulsively on the sheets.

'Mese, *ayezush*. That was your baby's head you felt. It's almost finished. Now breathe. With the next contraction, the body will come.'

Sure enough, I could see as her abdomen changed shape, as the muscles contracted once more, forcing the baby ever further down. Meseret called out again, and into my hands came her son, accompanied by a rush of clear fluid.

I looked across at Atsede, a smile of relief and happiness on her face. Ehuty was ululating quietly, leaning forward to plant kisses on Meseret's cheeks, her eyelids, her forehead. Meseret looked exhausted, but as her hands loosened their grip on the sheets, and came down to meet mine, taking her child in them and guiding him to her breast, the smile lit up her eyes. I sighed happily, as amazed and awestruck by Meseret as I am by every woman who gives birth, and grateful that we had been able to be the ones to guide her through it. Atsede left her chair, and was murmuring quietly to Meseret and the new baby as we guided her onto the bed, the umbilical cord still reaching inside of her. Minutes later her placenta delivered, and I was surprised to see the thick vessels that came together to form the umbilical cord doing so not in the centre of the placenta, as we would expect, but right on the on the membranes themselves, a velamentous insertion. *Gosh*, I thought, motioning to Atsede to look, *we were lucky*. Atsede's eyes widened as she saw, and as I watched, her mouth moved in a familiar prayer as she crossed herself, giving thanks to Lourde Mariam for watching over Meseret and her baby.

Atsede would mutter that same prayer a month later, lying prone on the operating table as Dr Rita splashed iodine over her abdomen, preparing to trace the scar of Mesmora's cesarean with her scalpel once more. Unusually, we had argued on the day of her second son's birth. I had watched her contract through two nights, and the first tendrils of fear were making their way through me. She hadn't progressed at all, despite good contractions, and I wondered if there was a reason why. We had tried everything, from the roasted, pounded drink of *telba* seeds the Gurage women drink to encourage birth, to keeping her moving, changing positions, finding a rock to step up on to, and back off again. Mesmora and Raphael had joined that game with great enthusiasm, leaping as far as they could each time, laughing riotously as, inevitably, they tumbled into the mud on landing. When, on the second day, she agreed to come with me to the hospital, I had a feeling that I knew what Dr Rita would say. Atsede had now passed 42 weeks, had had good contractions for well over 24 hours, and had already had a caesarean that precluded some of the augmentation options. The baby's heartbeat had held steady through the night, a fact for which I was intensely grateful, but there was only so long her uterine muscles could hold that force without putting undue strain on the scar tissue. As the evening of the second day came, Dr Rita had come once more, just as I had heard the baby's heartrate slow down with the contraction, and not pick up again afterwards with the speed it had previously.

Atsede had agreed to go with Dr Rita into the operating theatre, at last. As she cut through the skin, and peeled back the peritoneum, she let out a low whistle.

'Peritoneum full of fluid, and lower segment very thinned out, no more than 1.5mm.' Atsede and I both understood what that meant. Fluid in the abdominal cavity was often seen with obstructed labour, a sign of hours of contractions, and the tiny depth of muscle left pointed towards this intervention coming just in time. As I looked over the drapes, not wanting to leave Atsede's side, but also needing reassurance that we had made the right decision, I could see what Dr Rita meant. Atsede's scar hadn't quite dehisced, but the paper-thin muscles were bulging outwards with the pressure of the amniotic sac. It reminded me of another operation, when I had stood opposite Dr Rita as her assistant. During that one she had pulled apart the abdominal muscles only to find the baby's feet sticking bizarrely out of the uterus, which had completely opened up along the densely knotted, fibrotic scar tissue of the previous incision. Amazingly there was no bleeding, and the dehiscence hadn't extended, so the baby was born healthy and well, and the mother, after agreeing to a bitubal ligation to ensure no further pregnancies, had recovered in days.

As Dr Rita had pressed her scalpel against Atsede's uterus, the cloying smell of chorioamnionitis was instant. 'Can you smell that?' she had asked, not waiting for a reply, knowing we certainly could. 'This was a good decision for you and your baby, Atsede. The chorioamnionitis has started. We will start you on metronidazole as well as ampicillin, I think, just to be sure.' Laughing, she lifted Atsede's second baby, also a boy, just above the surgical field. 'And such a short cord. So much going on, Atsede. This baby would never have come vaginally.'

Tears of gratitude slipped from Atsede's eyes. I understood completely. Hearing those words provided the reassurance we both needed. I hadn't forced her into a caesarean – no one could force Atsede into anything she didn't want – but I certainly hadn't tempered my words when telling her what I thought of her decision to delay. Her recovery from this caesarean seemed easier than it had been with Mesmora, or perhaps we just knew better how to manage it. With the antibiotics, regular pain relief, and Aster and I staying by her side, passing Natnael to her, supporting his head as he fed so she wouldn't have to, three days later she was at home. Raphael, Mesmora and I slept on a mattress at her side, making sure she had the time and space to rest, to recover. It took days before Natnael learnt to nurse from both sides, and a few weeks before she stopped taking paracetamol altogether, but sure enough, with every day that passed, Atsede could move more easily.

I shared the sadness I knew she felt about a second caesarean, knowing how much she had wanted a vaginal birth. But when she brought it up, I realised that far more than that, what I actually felt was relief. Even during just over a year at the hospital, I had seen all too often what happens when the midwives and surgeons aren't there in time, and I would never forget that it was one such case that led to Atsede and I opening the Clinic at all.

As I thought this, sitting at Atsede's side, picking gently at the white plaster that covered the healing incision, wondering whether to just rip it off quicky or to go more slowly, the memory of that day came rushing in. I was standing, my hands full of freshly laundered sheets still warm from the sunshine, in the doorway of the birth room, unable to formulate a single thought. The curtains that had been drawn around the end bed in an attempt to afford a little privacy were twitched back, revealing Atsede and Selam standing silently, along with the nurses from the general medical ward. I couldn't comprehend what I was seeing. The woman's ankles were already bound, and her wrists joined over her chest. The nurses had just finished wrapping the final length of bandage around her head to keep her mouth closed, and across her eyes to ensure the same. A sheet was taken from my silent arms and pulled over her, the bump of her unborn baby still clearly evident. I had hurried past her bed space just a few minutes before, rushing to the laundry to get linen so we could take a woman to theatre for an emergency caesarean. It was one of those days when we hadn't had a moment spare. Tansei had come from a health centre, very unwell, but seemingly stable. We had started her initial medication, were monitoring when we could, and were awaiting Dr Rita, currently in the midst of a tricky surgical case, to come up with a longer-term treatment plan. One of the cleaners, Lubaba, gently took the remaining laundry from my arms and gestured to the bedside, where I joined Atsede and Selam to bear witness to Tansei's final rites. Still at a loss for what to say, I looked to them, the questions there in my expression. As I reached to smooth the sheet over Tansei's arm, I inadvertently brushed her skin with my fingertips. She was cool. Far too cool for her death to have been very recent. How had this happened? *How had we not realised?*

A woman's body is a masterpiece of resilience, able to withstand extraordinary challenges and emerge victorious. In times of feast and of famine, of war and of peace, all the days of the week and all the seasons of the year, women give birth. But growing a life is physiologically difficult. The heart has to move half as much blood again around, the lungs breathe enough to make sure it's full of oxygen, the hormonal system ensure everything stays receptive. A healthy woman can make the necessary adjustments, give a little, with the smooth muscle fibres throughout her body relaxing in response to the progesterone, so the blood vessels widen fractionally, but just enough, and with her kidneys picking up the pace to clean not only her own blood, but that of the baby, moved between them by the miracle that is the placenta. Then there is the demand of labour, the bunching of the thick, powerful uterine muscles, the passage of the baby through the pelvis, the inevitable blood loss that accompanies any birth, the attempts of the body to heal. A healthy woman can manage all of this, but a woman whose body had been ravaged by unchecked, untreated AIDS never stood a chance. Had she been able to access care, were a health facility closer, if she'd had a little money, the nurses and midwives could have counselled her through choosing a birth control option, allowing her to start the necessary antiretrovirals that may then have helped rein in her HIV. But she hadn't. And now the only release for her battered, exhausted body was to take her final breaths.

No other case, no other surgery or trauma or death, left a mark as deep as that of Tansei. To me, it was unforgivable that she had died alone, unnoticed. Having too few midwives and too many women is little excuse. Dr Rita saw my distress, and offered her benediction. Tansei had been deeply unconscious from the moment she was brought in; nothing we could have done would have made a difference. Her deep reflexes were depressed so she wasn't aware of the storm. But the turmoil I felt didn't abate. I lashed out at Atsede and Selam, as we often do to those closest to us who we know understand our pain and will forgive it, asking how they had let this happen. I flung the words at them, even though I knew, like me, that all morning they had been running between the theatre, the antenatal women and the emergency room, standing still only long enough to catch one of the many babies who chose today to arrive.

I saw that the look in their eyes was the same as the look in mine: regret and anger that these were the circumstances we were working in, that so many midwives around the world were working in, that led to a young woman dying without anyone bearing witness. Even if we couldn't have changed the ending of her story, we could have been there for the final chapter. They were just as affected as me and Tansei's death marked a turning point. From that moment on, Atsede and I were caught up in an idea, a dream, which we discussed endlessly, whether stirring the big pot of *wot* over the fire, or sitting writing notes at the desk in the hospital. It captured our interest to the exclusion of almost everything else. We would open a birth centre, where every woman matters, every woman is seen. Without the demands of such a high number of patients, we could give each woman the time and care needed for a positive and empowering birth. And so came months of planning, of meetings with the village elders, of persuasion and encouragement, gathering the wood and stones and mud needed to make our building. There was a plot of land: it was ours if we could find the money to construct, equip, and stock what would become the only birth centre of its kind in the area.

My parents, to whom I owe a debt of gratitude beyond words, were there, helping however and wherever they could, with breakthroughs coming in our formal registration as a charitable body with the UK Charity Commission, and in the participation of our newly-opened Clinic in well-recognised research projects.

My friends and family, midwives I'd worked with and trained with: everyone stepped up in a way far beyond what I had hoped for. We needed the calibre of Atsede's standing in the community to put our plan into action, and now we needed my access to potential funding to finish it. A stroke of serendipity saw us secure the support of the inimitable Australian doula Angela Gallo, a firework of a woman and a force to be reckoned with, willing to give so much and do so much. With her, our Clinic came to life. Quicker than we could have hoped, the panes of glass were in the windows, the tiles on the floor, and we opened the gates. It would be many months before we had access to electricity or running water, making do in the meantime with what we had, but the trees grew and the flowers blossomed, and before long the Clinic became the peaceful, beautiful space we had envisaged.

And the women came, not only from our town but from the surrounding villages. The drums beat loudly, and word of what we were doing got around. The support continued to pour in from all over the world. Over the coming months, we would welcome visitors from America, Australia, Norway, Italy and India, and to this day it is a place that echoes with laughter, a place of happiness and compassion and love, and, often, new life. As we came to understand the needs of the families we served better, we saw more and more the need for healthcare to be embedded within the community. For decades Ethiopia had been receiving foreign aid, billions of pounds and dollars poured into health development projects, and yet still the rates of maternal mortality and morbidity were among the highest in the world. The beginnings of a way to combat this came to light in our small corner of the country, and the quiet, unassuming support of Ethiopiaid UK took a chance in supporting the vision of the Clinic even as we were still trying to define it ourselves. We were able to implement new programmes of health delivery, which saw the Clinic midwives and nurses spend their days sitting among the men and women of the villages, just talking, sometimes with posters or aids that had everyone laughing, sometimes with cups of *kawa*.

While only Atsede and I know of its meaning, there is a small bird painted over the light switch on the wall of the Maternal and Child Health Room. Inspired by the butterflies and starfish we had strung across the windows of the Neonatal Unit at the hospital all those months before, which were the reminders of hope and perseverance and triumphing over adversity, the purple and pink bird has feathers that match the colours of the dress Tensai wore on the day we weren't there for her. I look at it every time I walk into the room, and often catch Atsede brushing her fingers across it. The bird has become a talisman of sorts, a protector for our women. And in the almost three years since we stood proudly by as the first baby was born, into his aunt's hands, to a mother kneeling on the floor, our guardian bird has seen hundreds of women, and thousands of patients, through the doors of the Clinic.

That first birth, a beautiful boy born to Genet, could not have been any more different from what I had become accustomed to seeing at the hospital. As much as the joy of watching Genet move as she wished, be surrounded by whoever she wished, birth in whatever position she wished, it was also the privilege of watching Atsede as a midwife under these circumstances. Without the pressures of managing the often-hectic Delivery Room at the hospital, and the sheer volume of women accessing the services there, her years of experience and deep understanding of birth were given a platform to blossom. She has coaxed and guided women through the pain of contractions, encouraged and heartened tired bodies and tired minds to keep going, and celebrated the extraordinary, ordinary moment of birth as if she were every woman's closest sister. With her by their side, the women were able to reframe their fears, reclaim their past difficulties, and walk away from birth empowered and grateful. Alongside her, I learnt to do this too.

Atsede

My mind was on Birtukan as Indie and I walked back across the grasslands from Wordena. The death of a child is a heavy burden to bear. Like the firewood bound by vines or the water in the yellow jerrycans, so many women here carry the weight of it every day. The men feel it too. Everyone does. I glanced back to see Indie throw a handful of grass seeds high into the air, watching them twist and spin in the breeze, and as I reach for a handful of my own, I smile, remembering Emar, my mother's mother. Indie spoke up.

'What will happen to Birtukan?' At Indie's question, I remember the empty eyes of the bereft mother as she stared into nothingness, unable to understand how, or why, her beloved son was gone. The loss of a loved one is always there, like light just catching the edge of your vision, or the words to a song you can't quite remember. After a time, it isn't sadness that comes with that, but a comfort, and you realise it isn't the loss you felt that's still there, it's the love. Until you reach that realisation, though, it is a difficult path, with much darkness. I think back to the *luxor* of my father, when friends and family slept under blankets and the stars because the *sahrbet* huts ringing the garden were full. The background sounds of soft conversation, of wood being chopped, and of *kawa,* coffee, beans being pounded were, in time, a balm to my family's anguished hearts. Remembering that Indie had asked me a question, I told her that Birtukan would be okay again one day, and that the village would be there to help bring her back from the edge until then.

As I made my way through the slim trunks of the towering eucalyptus, I heard Indie pause behind me. Turning, and smiling at her endless curiosity, I raised an eyebrow, waiting for the question.

'Atse, who is this *wog*?' I hadn't even realised I'd talked about him, so was surprised by the question. But it was an easy one to answer, so I turned back to our path as I explained.

'He's the guardian of Gurage knowledge. He knows everything about our culture. And he tells people what to do if they have stepped out of the Gurage ways.' I glance back over my shoulder to see Indie flicking a leaf between her fingers, thinking about my answer. I follow her lead, plucking a slim silver leaf from a low-lying branch. I find it difficult to put into words the role of the *wog*. He's a real person, but also mythical, not more than a man, but aside from that altogether. He knows everything, and sees everything. If we are uncertain about how to handle a situation as a Gurage, the *wog* can tell us. He sees solutions to problems that no one else can, all within the understood parameters of what is acceptable within our culture. I twirl the leaf again, as we continue to walk through the dappled shade back to the track where, I hoped, a *bajaj* would be waiting, able to take us back to the Clinic and the women waiting to be seen.

We sit now, hours later, in a comfortable silence, watching the flames and sparks dance against the backdrop of a starlit sky. I reached for a twig from our dwindling supply of firewood, and as I started peeling back the papery, brittle bark, the memories that I'd held back earlier in the day flooded in. Prominent among them all, the figure of my father, sitting by the doorway, ever present, wrapped in the rough-spun cotton *gabi*, his wrinkled, capable hands wrapped around the horsetail *chirra* in endless swishing movement in an attempt to keep the flies away. I remember him in the shade of the *sahrbet* thatch, a small glass filled to the brim with my mother's fiery *arakay* resting on his knee, watching us, his children, gambol like kittens in the sunshine, playing with sticks and stones and lengths of rope, in constant, effervescent motion. Then, when I was old enough to understand the challenges of raising a family without enough money, but young enough to dance off after the conversation without being too heavily weighed down, I sat at his side while he ate, and I remember him telling me that at night, when it was dark and cool in the shadowy depths of the hut, he would allow himself to sleep until 2am. Then, without fail, he would wake up to plan how he would spend every last *sentime* of his meagre salary, to decide which of his eight children would be able to have a new notebook for school, or a new pen, or a new bar of soap. In the thoughtless joy of youth, I'd tease him, asking how he knew it was 2am if we didn't have a clock, and it was only later that the magnitude of what he was saying sunk in.

The weight of responsibility always sat light on my father's shoulders; he wasn't one to rage against his fate, but accepted the challenges and triumphs of his life with a quiet stoicism. The days and weeks when we had nothing but a few handfuls of *gomen* greens to eat, dipped in a sauce of hot *mitmita* spice and water, and the months and years we spent barefoot dressed in worn-out, too-big clothes, melted away in the warmth of the boisterous laughter and unwavering love of a family who would survive it all.

The clatter of wood broke my reverie, and I looked around, blinking, at Indie, who had dropped several new branches onto the remaining bits of broken wood. She smiled proudly at her gatherings, sparkling eyes catching the light of the fire. I hadn't even heard her go; my heart and mind were years away in my memories, and it took a long moment to dispel the nostalgia. With a huge yawn, Indie jostled me. 'Come back, Atse. Meseret is almost there!'

'I'm not even going to ask where you found the wood. But I hope you were careful of the *gwencha*, the hyenas.' A shudder went through Indie as she gritted her teeth. I knew she hated the hyenas that prowled the edges of the town, scavenging the skins and bones of animals slaughtered by families at the times of festivals and feasts.

'Ha,' came her only reply, 'those hyenas. I'm not scared. No problem.' But by now, Indie had seen enough of the injuries inflicted by sharp teeth, and the immense strength of the jaws and forequarters behind them, young children snatched while playing in the dusky sunlight, and even once, from the back of the young mother carrying him. Fortunately, those she had seen had survived, but even when the bites are healing, the infections that come with filthy teeth are often just as bad. The hyenas didn't unnerve me in the same was as they did Indie, who disliked everything from their whooping cackle to their scruffy hides, but then I grew up with their presence always in the shadows. The most fundamental lesson taught as soon as a child can walk is that they never, ever go outside at night. The youngest children are told about the *amor* that lurk there, mysterious, dangerous fiends that will eat them, but as they get older and understand, the make-believe *amor* become less frightening than the real hyenas. Those living in the forest near our huts have grown ever more confident over the years, picking off goats, calves, chickens, even puppies after one of the dogs whelped in the shade of the roses growing around the wooden fence demarcating my father's land. Despite the threats and angry words hurled at them, there was nothing to be done. It isn't in our culture to deliberately kill an animal for anything other than food, even a hyena, for doing so would result in its pack taking revenge and wreaking havoc. Instead, we had a set of progressively bigger, thicker, heavier branches to brandish, and a metal can to thwack it against on the rare occasion a foray out into the dark *enset* was necessary. And the children learn to keep eyes peeled and stones in hand, in case they see one coming.

'Anyway, Atse, you know the hyenas around here are now caught up with their cubs!' Indie said, laughter in her voice. I smiled back, pleased she had remembered the folklore from earlier in the day, when the light rain broke through weak sunshine, and the nurses explained that when this happens, it means the hyenas are giving birth.

'Or maybe', I replied, grinning now, 'they are off searching for the gold from the lepers at the end of the rainbow!'

The laugh that had been there all this time suddenly bubbled out of Indie. 'Leprechauns!!! Atse leprechauns, not lepers.'

As if we'd summoned him, the low whoop of a hyena echoed through the night, followed a moment later by the groans of a woman about to birth her baby. Sure enough, as I shifted in the chair, stretching muscles cramped from sitting, Meseret's sister appeared through the door kept ajar.

'She'd like you to come in, now.'

I glanced at Indie, brushing bits of sawdust from her arms and still laughing to herself about the leprechauns, whatever they are. After a traumatic experience with her first son, resulting in a caesarean following an unsuccessful, and painful, attempt at delivering her child with a metal-capped vacuum, despite her pleas for the midwife to stop, Meseret had sought out our care for this baby for the simple reason that she was told we would listen to her.

Meeting her for the first time, four months ago, I could see the shadows in her eyes. She was afraid of what would happen. I had spoken to her until the shadows started to fade, shown her around the Clinic, delighted as she smiled at Mesmora and Raphael playing catch with the birthing ball before disappearing out of the door, giggling mischievously, and without the slightest hint of remorse, in response to my reprimands.

'Mese, beautiful sunsets need cloudy skies. The birth of this . baby doesn't have to be like your first. You don't need to be afraid. Would you like to meet Indie? She and I work together during the births, so she'll be here as well.' Meseret had nodded, shyly, and sat down in the chair I indicated. 'I'll go and find her.'

I leant out of the door, looking for Indie, wondering where the boys had gone to cause havoc now. I heard a shriek of delight from just outside the compound, and suspected I had my answer to both. Sure enough, as I rounded the sandstone corner, I saw them. Indie was sitting cross-legged on the grass, with Mesmora and Raphael crouched in front of her, heads bowed, looking at something in her hand with great concentration. The shriek came again as Mesmora jumped out the way of Indie's moving hand. Laughter soon followed. Reaching them, I saw why. Cupped in Indie's hand was a little, bright green treefrog. She looked up and caught my eye, offering her prize with a smile.

'*Kwuncha,* Atse?' A grin identical to that of the boys was etched on her face, well aware of the fact that I did not like frogs. As children, we were taught they had teeth and would bite, and no matter how many times Indie had assured me that wasn't true, I just didn't believe her.

'Oh, you are not funny, Indie. Leave the *kwuncha* alone, that poor thing, and come with me. I've got someone I want you to meet.' After placing the frog on the spreading leaf of the avocado tree, out of the reach of the boys but low enough down that they could continue to watch it, Indie came to my side.

'Moya, Raf, look after my frog, okay? We'll take him back to the house, so mummy Atse can keep him.' Laughing, she batted away the hand I had raised to swat her, and we watched the retreating backs of our young sons, who had just seen Yordannos coming down the track from school, and were keen to meet the playmate they adored, no doubt to show her the frog.

Meseret had met Indie that afternoon and had agreed to come to the Clinic for her birth, rather than stay at home, but asked that we gave her the space she needed throughout her labour to come to terms with the trauma of her first. Indie had spoken to her softly, reassuringly, agreeing in principle, but outlining the reasons why, every so often, she felt it would be better if we could check on her and the baby. A compromise was reached, one we were all happy with, and we became her midwives. Now, months later, the time had come for us to live up to our promises.

Throwing the last bits of bark into the firepit, I took the hand Indie had held out to help me, knowing that the bump of my second baby made it more difficult to stand up these days. As Meseret had wanted, Indie and I had spent most of the evening by the fire, drinking *chai* and eating *kollo*. As the hours passed, Indie would stand and move to the door, kept slightly ajar, more and more often. Cocking her head, she would listen to the sounds of Meseret's labour, judging the frequency, the strength, nodding with satisfaction as the contractions lasted longer, with fewer minutes in between. Every half an hour, she would open the door just enough to slip inside, waiting for a contraction to finish so she could hold the doppler to Meseret's *den* and find her baby's heartbeat. Without turning on the lights, or speaking much at all, Indie would count the beats for the next minute, an indication of how well the baby was handling the pressures of the contracting uterus, then turn and leave again, so Meseret could continue with just her sister there, a quiet presence in the corner, sometimes singing hymns in a low, melodic voice, sometimes with her hand on the lower part of Meseret's back. At the fireside once more, the air of controlled calm that Indie adopted around Meseret slipped as our conversation picked up again. Now, with midnight come and gone, it was almost time.

'Atse, why didn't you go home with the boys earlier? You know I could have looked after Meseret. You should be resting.'

'*Ende,* Indie, you know as well as I do, I'll get far more rest here than at home with those mad boys!' Chuckling in agreement she pulled me up, and we edged around the crackling flames and into the Birth Room.

Meseret was sitting on the ball as we entered, arms leant forwards over the bed, head resting in the crook of her elbow. She was naked, save for the thick white *gabi* draped over her shoulders. I raised an eye at Indie, who looked back with a smug smile, mouthing *told you so* in my direction. It had been a point of great debate, the blue ball that Indie had brought from England a few months ago. She insisted it was the perfect place for women in labour to sit, but I couldn't understand how they would stay steady enough to not fall off. Tonight, as I watched Meseret slowly rock her hips, and so the ball, from side to side, it appeared Indie was right.

As the contraction grew stronger, Meseret's groans deepened. Her sister came through the door behind us, whispering quietly. 'She said it feels like she needs to go to the *shintebet,* the toilet, but I remembered from my birth, that is how it felt when the baby was coming, so I said maybe you should come in first.'

I smiled at her, reaching out to lay a hand on her shoulder, 'Ah, Ehuty, why didn't you tell us you were a midwife! I could still be resting by the fire.'

The older woman smiled back playfully, 'No no, Atsede, you are *hwetawra,* with two souls, pregnant, you must walk around sometimes. Sitting still is not good for you or the baby!'

'The midwife speaks again!' We laughed quietly as Indie knelt at Meseret's side. I couldn't make out what she was saying, but Meseret nodded and, holding on to the bed in front of her, lifted herself from the ball. Indie deftly moved it away and reached under the bed for the green pot that was kept there, slipping it under Meseret as she squatted down. Fishing in her pocket for a glove, a minute later Indie stood, the pot in hand, and made her way to the toilet next door.

As she passed us, she smiled. 'Lots of urine. You've been keeping her drinking, Ehuty, that's good. Now her bladder isn't in the way of that baby, let's see how we go.'

Minutes passed before Meseret stood once again, still leaning forward with her hands on the bed, but needing space beneath her. As another contraction came, the groan became louder. Indie was at her side, a birthing sheet spread on the floor between them. On the stool next to the bed, Indie had opened the aluminium tin taken from the autoclave that morning. I looked at it, thinking of all the times in the last decade that I had opened similar tins. The many times, as well, that there were no tins to open, and I had to make do with whatever I could find. One memorable night, a story I tell too often according to Indie, there were sixteen births, and I was the only midwife there. Sixteen women, seventeen babies. I ran out of instruments after the first seven. Out of medication after 10. No one anticipated that there would be so many in one night. I moved from bedside to bedside, cleaning beds with one hand as I checked a baby's heartbeat with another. By morning, I was so tired I could barely lift my feet for the walk through the forest home. But the women had their babies. Aware of the circumstances of their labour, when I came back the following evening, I found every one of the sixteen women still there, waiting. They pressed baskets of eggs, jars of honey, rounds of bread wrapped in *enset* leaves into my hands as they murmured prayers, blessings, and thanks. Their gratitude moved me to tears. I was overwhelmed, and deeply grateful, that despite everything, each woman had felt cared for.

Another contraction came, and Meseret raised herself up on her toes, hands curling into the sheet in front of her, eyes closed and teeth clenched as she bore down.

'Good, good. Meseret, *anbessa*, lioness, good.' Indie was quietly reassuring her. I shifted the chair from the desk to face the birth, and sat down, leaning forward, watching. Meseret's sister moved up to stand on the other side of the bed, opposite her. She took up the chant.

'Good, Meseret, good.'

Continuing to groan loudly, the sweat beading on her forehead now running in rivulets either side of her nose and on to her chest, Meseret breathed heavily.

'Good, my sister, *anbessa*.'

Suddenly, Meseret cried out, Indie's gloved hands coming up between her legs as she did so.

'Meseret, that is your baby's head', Indie spoke, 'That's what you felt. Now breathe. With the next contraction, their body will come, too.'

Even as she spoke, the ripple hardened across Meseret's body, and with one final effort her baby was born. Meseret's sister began the ululating cry of congratulations and bent forward to shower her in kisses. Indie, grinning, passed the baby up to Meseret, then reached around the new mother to take the *gabi* from where it had been placed hanging on the IV stand, and wrapped it around them.

'*Enkuan des alesh,* Meseret! *Enuan des alesh,* Ehuty.' Laughter ricocheted around the room as Meseret turned gingerly to sit on the bed.

'A boy!' Meseret's sister called out as she lifted the corner of the *gabi,* helping Meseret move him to sit more comfortably in her arms. I stood up to join them, looking down at the slowly blinking eyes of Meseret's son. He was tiny, with wrinkled skin and fists clenched, but with a good colour and already trying to find Meseret's nipple to nurse. Meseret watched him with such tenderness, moving him a little to help, pulling the *gabi* around them more closely. There was no one else in the world who mattered at that moment.

It reminded me so strongly of holding Mesmora in my arms for the first time that I felt the tears form in the corner of my eyes, unbidden. He had also been tiny, just 2kg, and although his birth had been so very different from Meseret's, this moment, of a mother meeting her son, was exactly the same. My hand went to my own stomach, feeling the life within moving, wondering if my next birth would be like Meseret's, wondering if my baby was a boy or a girl.

One month from then, to the day I realised later, after nights of my contractions coming and going, I would have the answer. The birth of Natnael, like his older brother, was assisted by the quick hands and flashing scalpel of Dr Rita. Sometimes I felt sad that I would never know a vaginal birth, never experience the first test of motherhood. I voiced that one night, as I sat with Indie on the side of my bed, her hands on my swollen breast, moving rhythmically towards the nipple, catching the streams of milk in a small *sini*. Like Mesmora, Natnael was struggling to latch on to one side, leaving my breast full and aching. The relief that came as Indie expressed was instant. We would continue this, Natnael nursing on one side, Indie expressing the other, every few hours for the next five days. Each time, after Indie loosened the milk, I would lift Natnael to try. Then one day, no different from any other, he simply opened his mouth and latched on. The cry of triumph and surprise I let out summoned Indie to my side a moment later. She had thrown open the door, looking wildly around, an onion she was preparing for dinner still half-peeled in her hand, trying to work out what was wrong, until her eyes focused on the baby I now held nursing.

'He did it! Natnael, you wonderful baby!' She had danced around the room, as delighted as I was. 'And so much faster than your brother!' she added, scooping up Mesmora as he and Raphael burst into the room after her, little wooden cars in one hand and stones in the other, having left whatever game they were playing to see what all the fuss was about. Raphael looked at his mother, laughing with Mesmora, and held up his hands to join in. Bending down to lift them both, Indie continued to dance, declaring our sons were the cleverest there had ever been, and were sure to grow into the strongest and bravest. Laughing, she set the boys down, shoving them out the door in front of her, before turning around to smile at me. Later that night, when the boys were sleeping on the mattress on the floor, blankets flung aside in the heat, and Natnael, having just finished nursing, was lying contentedly next to me, eyes open but lids starting to grow heavy, Indie was once again sitting at my side. This time, she was peeling off the white bandage that protected the incision Dr Rita had made. Dithering about whether to just rip it off quickly, or peel it back bit by bit, I mentioned again my vague feeling being of disheartened at having had a second operative delivery.

'Oh Atse,' Indie had begun, her finger stilling at the edge of the plaster she'd started to try to pick at, 'you shouldn't think like this. How Mesmora, and Naty, came into the world is just one small moment in the journey. It isn't even the start, that was all those months you held them inside of you, nourishing them, and it certainly wasn't the end. You might not see why at the moment, but I am so thankful you had an operation. Not only because now I get to watch Mesmora and Natnael grow up, but also because you are still here with me. I don't even want to think how different this story might have been if we weren't in the time and place we are, Atse.'

I glanced at my youngest beside me, then over Indie's shoulders to our sons on the floor. While neither of my caesareans had really been an emergency, there was truth in what she had said. Especially with Natnael, given the diagnosis of chorioamnionitis, an infection in the membranes that held the amniotic fluid. Five days of strong antibiotics following the operation, flushed into my veins by Indie who rarely left my side, except to bring Mesmora and Raphael to meet the new baby, stopped the infection from spreading through my body, wreaking havoc wherever it went, but without either intervention, it could have been a very different story. I'd certainly seen enough of the alternate endings in the last decade to know it takes just one moment, just one decision, for everything to change. That was why Indie and I were sitting as we were right now, because of one moment, three years ago.

I know the day is as etched into Indie's memory as it is into mine, and Selam's too. To have a woman die in your care is a wrenching experience, one I have had to navigate too often, but having it happen without you realising is a different kind of heartbreak. The words of comfort that Dr Rita had tried to speak, that no one in the world could have saved Tensai, did little to assuage the sadness and guilt we felt. And yet, without her death, it is difficult to know if we would have thought of opening the Clinic at all, and even if we had, whether we would have pursued that dream with the single-minded determination that carried us through the bureaucracy, the setbacks, the indeterminate meetings and paperwork. In Indie and I together, we found the perfect combination. I had been the only midwife for so long that most people know me. In the markets and churches, on buses and *bajaj*, I see the babies born into my hands. We needed that reputation, my reputation, to encourage women to come to us. But we also needed Indie's ability to bring our vision to life through her impassioned words, and use that to marshal funds. One of us alone could never have opened the Clinic, and yet together, even from the earliest days of planning, it seemed infinitely achievable. Far faster than either of us could ever have imagined, we were waking in the morning to walk the track from the house we lived in together to the Clinic we opened together.

Every time a woman walks through the doors into the birth room, I catch myself reaching out to the small bird painted over the light switch. Tensai's bird. A reminder of how what we do came about, and why what we do matters.

About the authors

Indie McDowell is a classically trained anthropologist and a clinically trained midwife. Graduating first from the University of Cambridge, she then spent time working in Kyrgyzstan with UNICEF's Maternal and Neonatal Health Team before returning to the UK to complete her midwifery training. Following that, Indie took up positions in Cambodia and Malawi before finally settling in Ethiopia. After a year and a half running the neonatal services and the emergency obstetric response at a busy referral hospital in the rural south-west of the country with Atsede, they chose instead to open their own clinic, where compassionate and women-centred care could take centre stage.

Atsede Kidane is a Gurage midwife with over a decade of experience dedicated to the women of Cheha Woreda. She grew up a stone's throw from the hospital where she would later become the senior midwife, catching almost 10,000 babies and intervening in countless emergencies, touching many lives. She is a much-loved and well-respected member of the community, with women walking for hours to see her. After running the delivery room at the busy referral hospital, Atsede took up a post leading maternity services at a government-run health centre to try to improve the maternity services before coming together with Indie to open their own birth centre. Atsede was awarded the International Midwife of the Year Award in 2019, a tribute to her love of her profession and her passion for working to right the wrongs of health inequalities.

Acknowledgements

To the families of Gubrye and Cheha Woreda, for believing we wanted to help you, and allowing us to. To the staff of the Clinic, for wanting to work with us, and for always stepping up when we asked you to. To the clinicians and staff of Attat, for all you taught us, thank you. To Sr Rita and Sr Toni, for teaching us of faith and selfless service, thank you. To Sr Inge, Sr Florence, Sr Elaine, Sr Carol, Sr Nigist and Sr Elise, for the stories you told and the patients you served. To Ethiopiaid UK and GreenLamp, for the incredible work you do for the people of Ethiopia. To the Trustees of the Friends of AIC, for all the work behind the scenes that it took to register as a CIO. To the Pignatelli Trust, the Burdett Trust for Nursing, the Eleanor Rathbone Trust and the Souter Trust, for funding programmes run by the Clinic. To Pigeon Organics, Munchkin and Bear, Little Frog, Little Blooms, Codex Anatomicus, Clay

Bear, CUB, for the many wonderful donations. To the Roweth and the Harding families, for your generosity, and for thinking of us when there are so many amazing charities to consider. To Angel, Eva Rose, Sheena and Cheryl for your unwavering support. To Frankie, for your beautiful illustrations that capture so much of what we are lucky enough to see every day. To Laura and Olivia from United Agents, the first to hear our ideas and suggest how to form them into this book. To Martin, Zoë, Susan, Maria, and the team at Pinter & Martin, for making this book a possibility, and then a reality.

And lastly, to those who have given so generously over the years, and allowed the Clinic to continue to stay open. We think of each and every one of you often, and with the deepest gratitude.

Indie

To Will, my brother, for always having a ridiculous story to tell. To my grandparents, for reading my letters, and always replying. To Kirsten, Rachael, and Tory, for the laughter, thank you. To Lisa, Jenny, Tracey, Becky, Sarah and Di, who first showed what it means to be midwives, thank you. To Siany and Callum, for always being there, thank you. To Diego, you can open the last page now.

Atsede

To Aklila, Tadessa, Mekdes, Aster, Seyoum, Woinshet, Tamru, my brothers and sisters, thank you. To Asnakech, Aklila, Fikre, Tsega, Birhane, Sr Filseta, and Abba who became them too, thank you. To Hana, who shared so much of my midwifery journey. Tsehay, Pedros, Tisgey, Marta, Wolde, and Solomon *gashe* thank you. To Geremew, Bizunesh, and Tsigey, thank you. To Dawit, I could not have married a better man, thank you.

How you can help

Support the Atsede Clinic

Established in 2018, the Clinic serves a catchment area of 50,000 men, women, and children living in Cheha Woreda, predominantly in the town of Gubrye, but also the surrounding villages.

It was opened initially to provide maternal and children's health services, with an ethos of empowering women through compassionate and knowledgeable care during pregnancy and birth, and has since expanded to include an Emergency Room, as well as Laboratory and Pharmacy services.

The Clinic also coordinates a number of programmes aimed at re-embedding healthcare within the community, with an emphasis on responding to the needs identified by those accessing care, and initiating grass-roots projects.

Led by women, and staffed mostly by women, the importance of encouraging and supporting girls in the pursuit of education has also become an important aspect of the work of the Clinic, and there are now a number of scholarships and studentships offered for those who wish to work in healthcare.

The wellbeing of the Clinic staff sits at the heart of employment conditions. All those who wish to are enrolled in ongoing professional development courses, the children of all staff are supported through school, and salaries are paid well above the living wage.

The Clinic operates as a private NGO and a registered Ethiopian charity, relying on donations and grants to continue operations. Given that all of the Clinic staff grew up living well below the poverty line, and have experienced first-hand the challenges and difficulties of this, the Clinic charges the absolute minimum for some services in order to subsidise others, and offers free care to all those unable to meet costs.

For donations, which are always gratefully received, there are a number of options. The Clinic has an active JustGiving page (search The Midwives' Ambulance), currently raising funds to establish an obstetric and neonatal emergency ambulance service, which will be the first of its kind anywhere in Ethiopia. We are also supported by the UK charity, the Friends of AIC. The following bank details can be used for any donations.

Friends of AIC	*Atsede Kidane Zergaw*
CAF Bank	Commercial Bank of Ethiopia
Account No.: 00032675	SWIFT: CBETETAA
Sort Code: 40-52-40	Account No.: 1000271873526

More information on current projects can be found on the website, and to see more about the day-to-day goings on, follow @indiemidwife on Instagram.

www.atsedeclinic.com | @indiemidwife | indie.mcdowell@gmail.com | (+251) 0929 500894
Supported by UK Registered CIO Friends of AIC (118007)

Support Ethiopiaid UK

Vision: An Ethiopia in which every person has access to quality education, healthcare, and a life of dignity.

Mission: Breaking the cycle of poverty by enabling the poorest and most vulnerable and their communities to live with dignity, to build resilience, and achieve real and sustainable solutions to the challenges they face.

The Clinic, and Atsede and Indie, will always be so grateful to Ethiopiaid UK for believing in their vision, and their ability to achieve it, during the very early days. Without the support of Ethiopiaid UK, many of the outreach programmes, as well as the regular 'Circles' sessions held at the Clinic, would simply not have been possible. Not only the grant itself, but the confidence and trust placed in the Clinic, has had more of an impact that words can say.

Alongside the Clinic, Ethiopiaid UK support a huge range of projects and charities across Ethiopia, and have done so for decades. The most well-known of these, perhaps, is the Hamlin Fistula Hospital, the home of the late Drs Reg and Catherine Hamlin, who worked tirelessly throughout their lives to treat the women of Ethiopia suffering from childbirth fistulae. Alongside this important work, Ethiopiaid also maintains strong relationships with the APDA, The Cheshire Home for Disabled, and Wings of Healing, among many others. Each of these charities is well worth looking into further.

The Ethiopiaid approach is simple, and continues to be effective. Funds are raised for, and grants are given to, local Ethiopian partners to achieve lasting change and improve the lives of some of the country's poorest and most vulnerable communities.

Ethiopiaid focuses on the needs of vulnerable Ethiopians at grass-roots level. This hinges on sustainable relationships with trusted Ethiopian partners, who know the context and solutions. Partnerships continue as long as there's a clear need and opportunities to make lasting impact.

www.ethiopiaid.org.uk | @ethiopiaduk | lisa@ethiopiaid.org.uk | (+44) 01225 476 385
UK Registered CIO Ethiopiaid (802353)

Support GreenLamp

Education unlocks brighter futures, both for individuals and for entire communities. By sponsoring Ethiopian women to complete their midwifery training, GreenLamp has seen marked improvements in antenatal and intrapartum care in the facilities where these midwives go on to work.

Solar suitcases provide reliable lighting, communication, and power for rural delivery wards via sustainable, clean technology. The simple provision of facilities that most take for granted creates a safer, more dignified environment, and a measurable decrease in traumatic birth injuries.

The ripple effect of education and technology is incredibly powerful. Improved midwifery care reduces birth injuries that leave women stigmatised and isolated, while helping even just a few young women to access education creates community role models and leaders for the future.

www.greenlamp.ch | @greenlamp.ch

Support The Burdett Trust for Nursing

The Burdett Trust for Nursing is an independent charitable trust named after Sir Henry Burdett, the founder of the Royal National Pension Fund for Nurses (RNPFN). The Trust was set up in 2002 in recognition of the foundation, philosophy, and structure of the RNFPN. Nurses, midwives, and allied health professionals make up the majority of the healthcare workforce and play a pivotal role in the direct care to patients. The Trust makes grants in support of nurse-led projects, using its funds to empower nurses and make significant improvements to the patient care environment.

www.btfn.org.uk | @burdetttrust | administrator@btfn.org.uk | (+44) 0207 399 0102
UK Registered Charitable Trust The Burdett Trust for Nursing (1089849)

Support the Eleanor Rathbone Trust

The priority for the Eleanor Rathbone Trust is those charities supporting women, girls, young people, and families who are economically deprived and/or socially excluded. Internationally, the Eleanor Rathbone Trust supports projects delivered in sub-Saharan Africa, the Indian subcontinent, and projects in Palestine, or supporting Palestinian refugees.

www.eleanorrathbonetrust.org.uk | eleanorrathbonetrust@gmail.com
UK Registered Charitable Trust Miss E F Rathbone Charitable Trust (233241)

Also from Pinter & Martin

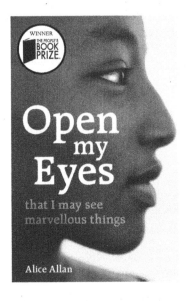

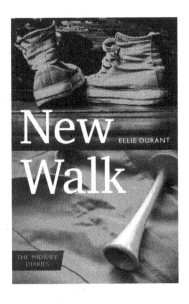

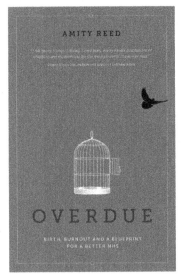

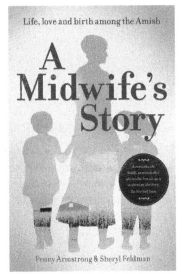